AF571816

Diagnosis and Treatment of Chronic Pain

Edited by

Nelson H. Hendler
Donlin M. Long
Thomas N. Wise

John Wright • PSG Inc
Boston Bristol London
1982

Library of Congress Cataloging in Publication Data
Main entry under title:

Diagnosis and treatment of chronic pain.

Bibliography: p.
Includes index.
1. Pain. I. Hendler, Nelson H. II. Long, Donlin. III. Wise, Thomas N. [DNLM:
1. Pain—Diagnosis. 2. Pain—Therapy.
WL 704 D536]
RB127.D53 616'.0472 82-4733
ISBN 0-7236-7011-0 AACR2

Published by:
John Wright • PSG Inc, 545 Great Road, Littleton, Massachusetts 01460, U.S.A.
John Wright & Sons Ltd, 42–44 Triangle West, Bristol BS8 1EX, England

Printed in Great Britain by
John Wright & Sons (Printing) Ltd. at The Stonebridge Press, Bristol

International Standard Book Number: 0-7236-7011-0

Library of Congress Catalog Card Number: 82-4733

For my parents, Winifred and Albert Hendler, and the new addition to my family, Lindsay, who joins Lee, Sam and Alex.

CONTRIBUTORS

Jerome D. Buxbaum, DDS
Associate Clinical Professor
Department of Physiology
The Myo-Oro-Facial Pain Clinic
University of Maryland
School of Dentistry
Baltimore, Maryland

Richard G. Black, MD
Associate Professor of Anesthesiology
Johns Hopkins University
School of Medicine
Baltimore, Maryland

James N. Campbell, MD, PhD
Assistant Professor of Neurosurgery
Johns Hopkins University
School of Medicine
Baltimore, Maryland

Cynthia A. Cimini, MS
Doctoral Graduate Student
Johns Hopkins University School of
Hygiene and Public Health
Baltimore, Maryland

Walter A. Hall
Research Associate
The Fairfax Hospital
Falls Church, Virginia

Nelson H. Hendler, MD, MS
Assistant Professor of Psychiatry
Assistant Professor of Neurosurgery
in Psychiatry
Johns Hopkins University
School of Medicine
Psychiatric Consultant to the
Chronic Pain Treatment Center
Johns Hopkins Hospital
Baltimore, Maryland
Clinical Director
Mensana Clinic
Stevenson, Maryland

Alan S. Hymanson, MD
Cardiology Fellow
Tufts-New England Medical Center
Boston, Massachusetts

Andrew R. Klipper, MD
Co-Chief of Rheumatology
Franklin Square Hospital
Baltimore, Maryland
Chief of Rheumatology
St. Joseph Hospital
Towson, Maryland

A. Lewis Kolodny, MD
Co-Chief of Rheumatology
Franklin Square Hospital
Chief of Rheumatology
North Charles General Hospital
Baltimore, Maryland

Michael J. Kuhar, PhD
Professor of Neuroscience, Pharmacology and Psychiatry
Johns Hopkins University
School of Medicine
Baltimore, Maryland

Donlin M. Long, MD, PhD
Professor and Chairman
Department of Neurosurgery
Johns Hopkins University
School of Medicine
Director of the Chronic Pain Treatment Center
Johns Hopkins Hospital
Baltimore, Maryland

Robert H. McPherson, BD, MA
Chaplain
Wilford Hall
United States Air Force
Medical Center
Lackland Air Force Base, Texas

Gavril W. Pasternak, MD, PhD
Assistant Attending Neurologist
Memorial-Sloan Kettering Cancer
Center
Associate Professor of Neurology
Cornell University
School of Medicine
New York, New York

Jacques M. Quen, MD
Clinical Professor of Psychiatry
Associate Director, Section on the History of Psychiatry
New York Hospital—Cornell Medical Center
New York, New York

Milton Reder, MD
Associate Physician
Post-Graduate Hospital
New York, New York

Milton A. Reder, MD
Rheumatology Fellow
Boston University School of Medicine
Boston, Massachusetts

Jerome P. Reichmister, MD
Clinical Assistant Professor of Orthopedic Surgery
University of Maryland School of Medicine
Instructor of Orthopedic Surgery
Johns Hopkins University School of Medicine
Baltimore, Maryland

Marcel A. Reischer, MD
Adjunct Assistant Professor of Rehabilitation Medicine
Department of Rehabilitation
University of Maryland School of Medicine
Baltimore, Maryland

John Rybock, MD
Assistant Professor of Neurosurgery
Johns Hopkins University School of Medicine
Baltimore, Maryland

William G. Speed, III, MD
Associate Professor of Medicine
Johns Hopkins University School of Medicine
Baltimore, Maryland

Henry A. Spindler, MD
Assistant Professor of Rehabilitation Medicine
Department of Rehabilitation
University of Maryland School of Medicine
Baltimore, Maryland

Mary Cowan Viernstein, PhD
Assistant Professor of Psychology
Johns Hopkins University School of Medicine
Baltimore, Maryland

Thomas N. Wise, MD
Chairman
Department of Psychiatry
The Fairfax Hospital
Falls Church, Virginia
Associate Professor of Psychiatry and Medicine
Johns Hopkins University School of Medicine
Baltimore, Maryland
Professor of Psychiatry
Georgetown University Medical Center
Washington, DC

Otto Wong, ScD
Director of Biostatistics
Environmental Health Associates
Berkeley, California

David A. Zohn, MD
Chief, Department of Physical Medicine and Rehabilitation
National Hospital for Orthopedics and Rehabilitation
Arlington, Virginia

CONTENTS

Section VI **Management**

PREFACE

When we decided to assemble a book on the diagnosis and treatment of chronic pain, we thought it best to avoid an all-inclusive, encyclopedic, or textbook approach. Instead, we chose to assemble a practical volume, written by clinicians with an interest in chronic pain, who have a wealth of clinical experience. The volume was designed to focus on common complaints that are seen in the everyday practice of medicine, regardless of the specialty. In many instances, the authors have chosen not to reference their chapters, but merely provide selective readings. In others, the authors have felt obliged to document each of their statements, and extensive references appear. In four instances, the chapters are derived from lectures given at Mensana Clinic for a Contin uing Medical Education course on the differential diagnosis and treatment of headache. Despite the variety of styles and formats, the chapters do have similarities: they offer relevant material that has broad clinical applications (with one or two notable exceptions which provide a theoretical foundation).

We hope that this compendium will serve as a useful handbook for physicians involved with the diagnosis and treatment of chronic pain patients. Despite the obvious gaps evident in this volume, we feel the reader will be compensated by the relevance and practicality of the material that is included.

Nelson H. Hendler, MD, MS
Donlin M. Long, MD, PhD
Thomas N. Wise, MD

SECTION I
Psychological Background

1 The Four Stages of Pain

Nelson H. Hendler

One of the most common errors that one encounters when reading a multitude of articles about pain is the failure of some authors to make the distinction between acute and chronic pain. One of the first physicians to appreciate not only the psychological differences between acute and chronic pain, but also the anatomical differences, was John J. Bonica, MD. While at first this may seem inconceivable, upon further examination it is quite apparent that almost all of the various pain states as they progress into chronicity are bound to produce psychological changes, since the debilitating component of the experience of chronic pain only worsens with time. Some authors have described this psychological response in other chronic disease processes. However, chronic pain has never been considered a disease per se, since there are multiple etiologies to the complaint of chronic pain. Yet, if one examines chronic pain as a distinct symptom complex, it becomes quite apparent that a host of similarities emerge when comparing and contrasting the psychological states of people experiencing chronic pain, regardless of its etiology.

One of the early reports, which divided the psychological responses into four stages, was published by Hendler et al in 1977. While the stages are not rigidly drawn, it is quite possible for patients to manifest characteristics of one or more stages or, in fact, all stages. These stages seem to parallel the response to death and dying as described by Kubler-Ross, and, in fact, differ only in the acceptance phase. The concept does seem to serve as a useful framework upon which to build an understanding of the psychological components of chronic pain. When one begins to integrate the psychological as well as the anatomical considerations, a more broad-based framework and understanding for the symptom complex of chronic pain can be appreciated.

In order to understand abnormal responses, one must study the natural phenomenology of a disorder and establish baseline responses in normal subjects. For this reason, the material in this chapter is derived from studies of well-adjusted individuals, who, as the result of chronic pain, have developed psychological problems. Very often, this relationship is not fully appreciated, and psychiatrists and other physicians have the tendency to interpret psychological responses at any given time as the cause rather than the result of chronic pain. This has given rise to a variety of pejorative terms for chronic pain patients, including "lowback loser," the "pain-prone personality," the "pain neurosis," and others. The lack of sophistication and empathy demonstrated by the authors of these uncomplimentary epithets is understandable, since chronic pain patients can be incredibly demanding of a physician's time, and most trying of his or her patience. However, if one studies chronic pain patients in a longitudinal fashion and follows them during the course of their odyssey through chronic pain, it is quite apparent that in previously well-adjusted individuals personality changes occur as the result of chronic pain. For this reason, the remainder of the chapter is based on what one must term a normal response to chronic pain.

Premorbid Adjustment

When analyzing a patient's response to chronic pain, it is imperative to know what the person was like prior to the acquisition of the pain. Often, the prepain or premorbid adjustment lends a variety of clues which helps one understand how the patient deals with adversity, how stable the individual is, and how socially well-adjusted or maladjusted the individual is. In order to study a normal response to chronic pain in a well-adjusted individual, one must outline some of the criteria for establishing the fact that a patient was functioning well prior to the onset of chronic pain. To do so requires a thorough and extensive history of not only the social, but psychological, sexual, and financial adjustment the patient may or may not have made prior to his illness. In a well-adjusted individual, one finds the following features:

1. A good work record, with steady employment and progressive advancement up to the time of the onset of chronic pain.
2. A stable family background, with the absence of a history of alcoholism, child abuse, drug abuse, arrests, and suicide in family members.
3. A negative psychiatric history, with no previous suicide attempts, depressions, or consultations with psychiatrists prior to the onset of chronic pain.
4. The absence of prior use of narcotics, tranquilizers, hypnotic drugs, excessive alcohol intake, or commonly abused street drugs.
5. A good marital history, with marriage occurring between the ages of 20 and 30, and the absence of divorce or marital maladjustment prior to the onset of pain.
6. Lack of financial difficulties prior to the onset of pain.
7. A good sexual adjustment, with the absence of difficulty with orgasm (for both males and females) and erection (for males).
8. No difficulty sleeping prior to the onset of pain.
9. No radical changes in weight (more than 20 pounds' fluctuation) other than a conscious attempt to lose weight when it was medically indicated and appropriate.

Obviously, there are a host of other parameters that might be considered, but the above list touches on all major aspects of social, sexual, and marital adjustment. If a patient is free of difficulties in seven out of these nine categories, then one must safely assume that his prepain (premorbid) adjustment was good.

Acute Pain (first two months)

After the well-adjusted individual acquires pain, the initial stage is the acute phase. During this stage, the patient realistically expects that his pain will get better. During this stage of the pain, the patient may take narcotic analgesics for a brief (one to two weeks) period of time and may require no other medical intervention. Also, during this period of time, the patient manifests none of the psychological disturbances that one sees in later stages of pain other than occasional difficulty sleeping. The following tests should yield normal results when administered during this stage of the pain process.

1. MMPI (Minnesota Multiphasic Personality Inventory test), a 566-question test consisting of true or false answers and designed to assess personality traits.
2. SCL-90 (Symptom Check List), a 90-question test developed by the Johns Hopkins Hospital group headed by Dr. Leonard Derogatis and designed to measure changes in the psychological status of an individual over time.
3. The Hendler Screening Test for Chronic Back Pain (HPT) (if the patient has back or limb pain).

Anatomically, the various neural pathways for acute pain differ from those for chronic pain. In acute pain, the anatomical connections begin with the receptor sites in the periphery, whether it be visceral receptors or common skin receptors. These fibers impinge on the substantia gelatinosa of the spinal cord and enter at various levels. They then ascend in the spinal cord, carried by the neolateral spinal thalamic tract. They transverse the brain stem and do not send projections to the reticular-activating system, but rather synapse within the thalamus. Then, various relays and interconnections of the thalamic nuclei occur, and afterwards the message of pain is transmitted to several areas of the somatosensory cortex. It is here that the pain is perceived and the patient recognizes that he has pain.

Subacute Pain (two to six months)

By now, the pain is beginning to distress the patient. Both the MMPI and the SCL-90 tests reflect change. Elevation of scales 1 and 3 (hypochondriasis and hysteria, respectively) on the MMPI, representing the so-called conversion V seen in hysterical conversion reactions, indicate an emerging preoccupation with physical problems. Likewise, the SCL-90 reflects this concern, since SOM (somatization) and ANX (anxiety) scales are usually elevated. The Hendler Screening Test for Chronic Back Pain usually has scores between 15 and 20 during this stage which suggests that the patient has not yet begun to experience the depression chronic pain can bring. This stage corresponds to the denial stage of the dying patient, as outlined by Kubler-Ross, which occurs early in the chronic pain process. Since the patient is denying the prospect of chronic disability, there is no evidence of depression. The patient retains the hope that the pain and disability, ie “loss of a loved object,” will be resolved. Subtle changes in personality or behavior such as increased irritability, insomnia, being awakened from sleep by pain, social isolation, and the beginning of the use of analgesics and sleeping medications may take place.

The anatomical pathways of subacute pain are the same as those of acute pain.

Chronic Pain (six months to eight years)

At this time, even the previously stable patient begins to experience depression. The MMPI and SCL-90 tests begin to show the neurotic triad of elevated scales 1, 2, and 3 on the MMPI, and the SOM, obsessive compulsive, interpersonal sensitivity, DEP (depression), ANX (anxiety), and HOS (hostility) scales are elevated on the SCL-90. These changes indicate that the patient may have begun to have suicidal thoughts, may have stopped or reduced work secondary to the pain, and recognizes the possibility that the pain may persist. The depression alternates with feelings of anger and attempts at bargaining with physicians about pain relief ("just get rid of 50% of this pain") and corresponds with the advanced stages of a dying patient. Although this comparison may seem a bit extreme, both the pain patient and the dying patient have experienced losses, either of functioning or of hope, and are trying to learn to cope with the loss.

The pain patient by now is experiencing some trouble with the marriage, sexual activity is reduced, is beginning to feel like a burden, has lost some self-esteem, and asks "Why me?" The patient may be abusing narcotics and may have begun to "doctor shop"; in addition, the patient may have undergone several operative procedures and may have feelings of guilt. The sleep pattern is disturbed, with difficulty falling asleep resulting as much from anxiety and depression as from pain, and with awakening because of pain and depression being reported. There may be weight loss because of the reduced appetite that accompanies depression, or weight gain resulting from reduced exercise because of limitation secondary to pain. The patient reports hopeless and helpless feelings, which are classic manifestations of depression and anxiety.

As the patient progresses through the chronic stage, the depression begins to resolve. Since depression has been described as anger turned in on oneself, it is not surprising that as the depression lifts the patient becomes overtly hostile toward members of the family, physicians, and the employer. The anger may also be better understood if one examines the dynamics of dependency. Very often, chronic pain patients become reliant and dependent upon members of their family and physicians for assistance. Additionally, they may for a variety of reasons become dependent upon insurance carriers or employers for providing income during the period of time that they are disabled by pain. This fosters a sense of dependency, which, in normally independent individuals, is repugnant. In response to dependency, one normally refrains from expressing anger at the person on whom he is dependent, only because the fear of losing the support of the person outweighs the anger. Additionally, at this stage, the patient normally expresses a degree of jealousy and resentment of the person on whom he is dependent. Thus, the pent-up anger which was causing depression now explodes upon the scene, with a variety of appropriate and sometimes inappropriate outbursts. The resentment and jealousy that the patient may have felt toward family members who had been of assistance to him becomes very evident, and the fear of losing these family members is now replaced by months and years of repressed hostility. This is one of the most difficult stages for the chronic pain patients and for their family members.

After the anger has subsided, the patient then resorts to a substage of chronic pain which parallels the dying patient, bargaining. During this substage, the patient tries to negotiate with physicians for pain relief and with family members for assistance. Patients usually become somewhat contrite, since they have previously alienated a variety of acquaintances with their angry outbursts. It is during this stage that the patient tries to negotiate additional pain-relieving techniques with the physician, tries a variety of unproven treatments in an attempt to relieve the chronic pain problem, and begins to negotiate with family members about appropriate and inappropriate levels of assistance that they may require around the house. The patient's behavior becomes more rational, and consequently more functional. It is at this stage that the patient becomes more adept at negotiating with insurance carriers, workmen's compensation carriers, attorneys, and employers. It is the prodrome to entering into the final stage of chronic pain, the subchronic or acceptance stage.

The anatomy of chronic pain differs from that of acute and subacute pain for a variety of reasons. Initially, as in acute pain, the sensory input travels along nerve fibers from the viscera and the periphery. However, when these fibers reach the spinal cord, the information is carried in the paleolateral spinal thalamic tract, which is anatomically distinct from the neolateral spinal thalamic tract of acute or sharp pain. The fibers then ascend in the paleolateral spinal thalamic tract to the brain stem, where they send projections into the reticular-activating system. This pathway differs from that of acute pain, in which the ascending fibers do not send projections into the reticular-activating system. As the fibers carrying the message of chronic pain ascend into the brain, they also send projections into the hypothalamus, as well as the thalamus. Again, this is different from the fibers of acute pain, which send projections only to the thalamus. From the thalamus and hypothalamus, a variety of pain messages ascend into the somatosensory cortex and areas of the frontal lobe, where the sensation of chronic pain is perceived.

The most striking neuroanatomical distinction between acute and chronic pain is the involvement of the limbic system which occurs in chronic pain. The limbic system controls a variety of emotions through hypothalamic and temporal lobe interconnection. From a neurochemical viewpoint, the involvement of the hypothalamus and other parts of the limbic system is important, since the vast majority of the biogenic amine neurosynaptic transmitters, which control emotion and some of the perception of pain, are located within this discrete anatomical area. Also, the neurosynaptic transmitters involved in sleep, and the newly discovered enkephalins function as neurosynaptic transmitters within this area, which has been documented by the presence of morphine-like receptor sites that intermingle with other receptor sites for biogenic amines. A more detailed description of the neuroanatomy of this area is contained in Chapter 17, and the neurochemistry is more fully explained in Chapter 18.

Subchronic Pain (three to 12 or more years)

In this stage, the patient has "learned to live with the pain" but still does not accept it. In fact, the pain patient never accepts the pain and its attendant disability. In this way, the pain patient differs from the dying patient who seemingly becomes peaceful in the final acceptance of death. Unfortunately, the pain patient has an indeterminate sentence and a more chronic, long-term course. At this stage, the pain patient has discontinued narcotics, has changed jobs or is functioning at the old job with almost the same degree of efficiency; sexual activity has returned. Sleep is less disturbed, and the depression is resolved. The patient's marriage has either ended or consolidated. The MMPI test shows elevated scale 1 (hypochondriasis) while the SCL-90 test has elevated SOM scales; the depression scales are again low on the SCL-90, but may not have returned to normal on the MMPI because of the structure of its questions. The pain patient's faith in treatment is much less evangelical than in the earlier stages, and he is beginning to settle into a readjusted lifestyle that demands coping with the chronic pain.

The anatomy of subchronic pain is similar to that of chronic pain.

By reviewing the premorbid personality and the four stages of chronic pain, one can see that chronic pain patients actually undergo an arduous odyssey that carries them through the full range of human emotion. While this chapter has dealt primarily with the psychological response to chronic pain in a previously well-adjusted individual, many of the psychological features can be found superimposed upon preexisting personality disorders or neuroses. Patients suffering from both preexisting psychiatric disorders and reactive disorders secondary to chronic pain present one of the most difficult therapeutic challenges to all physicians involved in their care. However, it is most important to bear in mind that preexisting psychiatric disorders and the normal psychological response to chronic pain exist on two different and mutually exclusive axes, and require different modalities of treatment and intervention. This is in opposition to the abnormal or exaggerated response to chronic pain that only serves to worsen the preexisting personality disorder or neurotic axis. This conceptual framework will be more fully explained in the following chapter.

BIBLIOGRAPHY

Hendler N, Viernstein M, Gucer P, et al: A preoperative screening test for chronic back pain patients. *Psychosomatics* 1979;20:801–808.

Hendler N, Derogatis L, Avella J et al: EMG biofeedback in patients with chronic pain. *Dis Nerv Syst* 1977;38:505–509.

Hendler N, Fenton JA: *Coping with Chronic Pain.* New York, Clarkson Potter, 1979.

Hendler N: *Diagnosis and Nonsurgical Management of Chronic Pain.* New York, Raven Prcss, 1981.

Kübler-Ross E: *On Death and Dying.* New York, Macmillan Co, 1969.

2 Factors Determining Acute Pain Response

Thomas N. Wise
Walter A. Hall
Otto Wong

Pain is an elusive concept. Qualitative verbal descriptors are overly subjective and demonstrate great individual variability. As knowledge concerning the effects of noxious stimuli grows, the complexity of pain as a percept, a neuroanatomical entity, a biochemical phenomenon, or a stimulus for related instrumental behavior becomes apparent. Mersky[1] has examined the difficulties in defining pain and has settled upon the definition that pain "is an unpleasant experience which we primarily associate with tissue damage or describe in terms of such damage or both." Medical care is implicit in this definition since the concept of pain directs the uncomfortable individual to a medical delivery system.

Because pain is too global a concept, it must be qualitatively viewed as either an acute or chronic phenomenon. Recent data concerning psychological characteristics of pain patients often have come from individuals with chronic pain. Furthermore, pain clinics are primarily directed toward chronic debilitating complaints. Acute, self-limited pain has been studied in laboratory settings with volunteer subjects. Early clinical investigations also have helped elucidate vicissitudes of acute pain. Beecher's[2] observations of acute traumatic wounds on a battlefield demonstrated that the meaning of a situation could modify an individual's request for narcotic medication. Egbert et al[3] demonstrated that preoperative training in relaxation exercises modified postoperative narcotic utilization. Experimentally, Chapman and Feather[4] demonstrated dysphoric effects such as anxiety-potentiated experimental pain estimation. Thus, pain becomes a final common pathway between various personality styles, psychological states, and situational factors. The surgical situation provides an "in vivo" setting for further investigation of the relationship of psychological factors and the phenomenon of acute pain.

Methods

In order to investigate the relationship between individuals' cognitive styles, psychological status, and pain estimation and response, two separate surgical populations were utilized. Thirty-seven individuals consecutively scheduled for elective cholecystectomy were interviewed and followed postoperatively. Four of these individuals were not included in the results; two declined to fully cooperate and two did not speak English. Eleven men, aged 29 to 58 years, and 22 women, aged 27 to 75 years, participated. Demographic characteristics revealed these individuals to be solely from classes two and three of the Hollingshead two-factor socioeconomic scale. All the male subjects were married; within the female sample, 16 were married, two were divorced, two widowed, and two single. Each patient was interviewed on the day of admission. They were administered the brief version of the General Health Questionnaire (GHQ), a 30-item questionnaire designed to assess the presence of psychological illness, and the Symptom Check List (SCL-90), another multidimensional psychometric instrument.[5,6] Patients also completed the Embedded Figures Test to determine their degree of psychological differentiation and the Rotter Locus of Control Inventory to assess their internal-external orientation.[7,8] The GHQ documents whether an individual has a minor psychiatric illness. The definition of this illness is a level of anxiety or depression of such magnitude that the individual would benefit from outpatient psychological treatment. The SCL-90 measures the symptomatic status of an individual along nine dimensions. It documents the state, not necessarily the trait, level of depression, hostility, anxiety, obsessionalism, etc. Its absolute values are derived from comparison with normative populations. The Embedded Figures Test measures an individual's tendency to see a visual field in a global fashion or in a more analytic manner. Can he differentiate the forest from the trees? The test categorizes one as *more* or *less* differentiated. The differentiated person is more analytic and utilizes defenses of isolation and intellectualization. The global style concurs more with the defenses of denial and repression. This style might indicate how an individual reacts to somatic discomfort. Specifically, can the individual isolate the pain via distractions such as reading or viewing television, or does pain cast a total shadow over his subjective sense of function? The locus of control paradigm measures how vulnerable an individual is to external reinforcement. Does he respond to environmental influence or feel he has to do everything on his own, ie, even recover from surgery or cope with pain?

On the day following surgery, the patients were asked to assess their perception of pain utilizing a 100-mm visual analog scale. This scale is nothing more than a line 100 mm long on which a patient is asked to place a mark which represents the amount of pain he is feeling, with 0 mm being the equivalent of no pain, and 100 mm equaling the most intense pain the patient has ever experienced. This was done at 10:00 in the morning and 4:00 in the afternoon.[9] These twice daily analogs were administered until the patient was discharged. The amount of pain medication utilized, in equivalent units of 75 mg of meperidine, was noted. The total amount of narcotic used throughout the postoperative stay was then determined. Analysis of variance showed no significant differences between the men and women of the group in respect to age, marital status, prior surgery, pain medication utilized, or locus of control. The mean values for completing the Embedded Figures Test did differ; however, this result would be expected as there is a significant variance between genders in the psychological differentiation construct.[10] Statistical interpretation of the data utilized parametric tests that allowed inferential assessment of significant differences between the sample populations.

Results

Psychological status of group None of the 33 subjects examined satisfied Feighner and co-workers'[11] criteria for a diagnosable psychiatric illness. Twelve of the individuals (two men and ten women), however, were considered to have a psychological disturbance as measured by the General Health Questionnaire (GHQ).

Relationship of preoperative affective status to pain perception and utilization The sample was divided into those who scored 4 or above or less than 4 on the GHQ. The group identified as having a psychiatric illness as manifested by a GHQ score of 4 or more utilized significantly more pain medicine than the low scorers (see Table 2-1). No significant relationship was found between these two subsets of GHQ scorers and their perception of pain.

Table 2-1
General Psychological Status and Pain Medication

GHQ Score	N	Mean Amount of Medication (*Units of 75 mg Meperidine Doses)*
Equal to or greater than 4	12	29.67*
Less than 4	21	17.48

*$t = 2.17$, df 15, $p \leqslant .045$

Relationship of personality variables to pain perception and pain medication Correlation between degree of psychological differentiation, the tendency toward field dependence as measured by the Embedded Figures Test, and pain perception was significant for the total group (see Table 2-2). When partitioned by sex, the correlation showed statistical significance for the female subset only. Use of pain medication was not significantly correlated with degree of field dependence.

Table 2-2
Correlation between Psychological Differentiation and Pain*

N	Embedded Figures Test	Pain Medication	Pain Perception
33	Total group	.0778	.3526†
11	Men	.0411	−.2975
22	Women	−.2609	.4288‡

*Toward field dependency
†$p < .05$
‡$p < .01$

The relationship between internal-external locus of control and pain perception and tolerance did not reach statistical significance for the group as a whole or subgroups of men and women (see Table 2-3). The relationship between external control and pain perception in the subgroup of women did approach a significant level ($.06 < p < .10$).

Table 2-3
Correlation between Locus of Control and Pain*

N	Rotter *(I − E)**	Pain Perception	Pain Medication
33	Total group	−.1934	.0456
11	Men	.1917	.3266
22	Women	−.4018	−.0995

*Tendency toward external locus

Relationship of cognitive style to preoperative affective status A highly statistically significant correlation between the level of psychological differentiation and the degree of anxiety and depression as measured by the SCL-90 was found within the sample as a whole (see Table 2-4). When the group was partitioned by sex, the statistical significance was lost. The level of psychological differentiation did not correlate at a level of confidence with the General Health Questionnaire except when men were measured alone.

Table 2-4
Correlation between Cognitive Style and Psychological Status

N		Anxiety	Depression	SOM	GSI	GHQ
	Rotter*					
33	M + W	.1710	.3476§	.0468	.1867	.3077
11	M	.3760	.7263‖	.6656§	.7506‖	.4323
22	W	.0820	.2398	−.2175	−.0080	.2345
	EFT‡					
33	M + W	.4762‖	.6012¶	.3906§	.6818¶	.2666
11	M	.2974	.5851	.2919	.5515	.6663§
22	W	.1791	.3129	.2467	.4915§	−.1661

* Tendency toward external locus
‡ Toward field dependency
§ $p < .05$
‖ $p < .01$
¶ $p < .001$

The relationship of the locus of control to psychological status showed a statistically significant correlation between the group as a whole and the level of depression. This finding proved to be the case in the subset of men within the sample. There was no significant correlation, however, with the dimensions of anxiety or the General Health Questionnaire and locus of control.

In order to investigate the acute pain response in an individual with a chronic pain condition, the pain estimation and narcotic utilization of individuals undergoing back surgery were compared with the group undergoing cholecystectomy. The same methodology was utilized except that field dependence-independence was not measured. The comparison between the two groups revealed the following results.

Population characteristics The 33 individuals of each group were compared for demographic variables which are displayed in Table 2-5. No significant differences were noted for sex, mean age, or marital status. The previous surgical experience of both groups was similar. Twenty-five of the individuals with gallbladder disease had undergone general surgery with anesthesia, whereas, in the group with back pain 29 had experienced past surgical procedures. As spinal disease is often a sequelae of trauma, the series with back surgery was surveyed for pending litigation. Only three of the individuals within this group had utilized workmen's compensation.

Table 2-5
Demographic Variables

Variable	Patients with Back Pain	Patients with Gallbladder Disease	t or Chi Square Value
Age	Mean = 47.1	Mean = 44.9	$t = 0.790$, not significant
Sex	Male = 19 Female = 14	Male = 11 Female = 22	$\chi^2 = 2.994$, not significant
Marital status	Married = 30 Single, Widowed or Divorced = 3	Married = 27 Single, Widowed or Divorced = 6	$\chi^2 = 0.514$, not significant
Past surgery with anesthetic	Yes = 29 No = 4	Yes = 25 No = 8	$\chi^2 = 1.62$, not significant

Personality style The mean value for the locus of control as measured by Rotter's 23-item questionnaire was not significantly different for either the patients with back pain or gallbladder disease (see Table 2-6).

Preoperative affective status The patients with back pain voiced significantly more complaints in the somatization dimension than their counterparts with gallbladder disease (see Table 2-7). They were significantly more depressed than the other group with gallbladder disease, and their overall level of symptom distress was also significantly greater than the postcholecystectomy subjects. The level of anxiety experienced by both groups preoperatively was not significantly different.

Pain estimation and tolerance The two groups showed no significant difference in their estimation of pain as measured by visual analog scales (see Table 2-6). Patients with back pain, however, used significantly more medication than their postcholecystectomy counterparts.

Discussion

Elucidation of acute pain behavior suggests that preoperative emotional status, personality style, and pain estimation and response are interrelated.[12] This has been done in both experimental and actual pain situations. The methodologic difficulties of the experimental situation have been outlined by Graffenreid et al.[13] The surgical experience with postoperative pain provides a naturalistic setting for the study of pain response. The stress of surgery, however, must be considered as an important variable in any investigation. Davidson and Neufield[14] have demonstrated that pain response can be partitioned from the stress of surgery. This provides a sturdier connection between the independent variables of personality style, psychological status to the dependent factors of pain estimation, and narcotic utilization. Prior studies have utilized heterogeneous surgical populations. This creates methodologic problems because of differences between surgical procedures. Each of these procedures, cholecystectomy and back surgery (either cervical or lumbosacral) is generally done for relative indications.[15,16] Thus, psychological factors may play a part in the reporting of symptoms leading to surgical treatment.

Table 2-6
Pre- and Postoperation Variables

	Mean Value		
Variable	*Patients with Back Pain*	*Patients with Gallbladder Disease*	*t Value*
Somatization	1.065	0.646	3.4765, significant at 0.001 level
Obsessive-compulsive	0.758	0.527	1.7910, not significant
Interpersonal sensitivity	0.420	0.349	0.5400, not significant
Depression	0.832	0.546	2.0476, significant at 0.05 level
Anxiety	0.694	0.518	1.4047, not significant
Hostility	0.359	0.319	0.3628, not significant
Phobic anxiety	0.138	0.138	0, not significant
Paranoid ideation	0.262	0.263	0, not significant
Psychoticism	0.306	0.242	0.7812, not significant
GSI	0.549	0.393	1.8678, not significant
PSDI	1.593	1.332	2.4564, significant at 0.05 level
Rotter	8.606	6.939	1.3737, not significant
Pain medication	34.303	21.909	2.4504, significant at 0.05 level
Pain analogues	36.848	27.970	1.8043, not significant

Individual pain response is a complex interaction of cultural, social, and psychological factors.[17] Previous investigations have studied either situational affective states or persistent cognitive variables. The relationship between enduring personality styles, dysphoric emotional states, and pain responses remains ill defined. A previous report suggested that field independent characters experience lesser tolerance to a cold pressor stimulus.[18] Likewise, externally located individuals were thought to need more analgesics.[19] This investigation rejects earlier views of a simple relationship and supports a multifactorial approach to pain response. It supports Adler and Lemassy's[20] findings that a cognitive style is hindered by dysphoric affects which interfere with ability to cope with noxious stimuli. Their report demonstrated no correlation between pain tolerance and level of psychological differentiation. They utilized experimentally induced pain upon paid volunteers. Our study's population of postsurgical patients allowed for the noxious stimuli to be divided into individuals' magnitude estimation of discomfort and measurement of pain tolerance gauged by narcotic utilization. This might explain our results which differ from Adler's investigation. The amount of pain experienced as measured by individual analog scales was found to significantly correlate with increasing field dependence. The lack of correlation when the group was partitioned by sex might relate to the small numbers in the male and female subgroups. The cognitive variable of field dependence-independence denotes an individual's ability to globally or analytically perceive his environment whether it be internal bodily sensations or external stimuli.

Previous studies of this enduring trait suggest that less differentiated individuals, those who are field dependent, expect more environment support such as global information and structure from authority figures. The field independent subject has a more developed concept of his body and better developed psychological defense mechanisms than the field dependent individual.[21] Thus, it has been suggested that the more field independent individual would show increased vividness to perception to afferent somatesthetic impulses which would thereby give him less pain tolerance. Our present study suggests this might be an oversimplified impression. Field dependent individuals estimate a greater magnitude of pain but tolerate the same amount of noxious stimuli as their more psychologically differentiated counterparts. In previous experimental designs, patients are allowed to stop noxious stimuli whereas our study group had to endure their discomfort. This noxious stimuli could be divided between pain perception and pain tolerance. In addition to analgesic medication, environmental supports could mitigate discomfort. It is understandable that individuals who globally perceive their environment, whether bodily sensations or external stimuli, might be more uncomfortable. Yet, the lack of correlation with pain medication might be explained by the utilization of environmental supports from the physicians, nursing staff, and family by field dependent individuals in lieu of analgesics.

Although field dependency–independency by itself was not a significant variable in pain medication, affective status was. Less differentiated individuals were significantly more anxious and depressed. These dysphoric affects were positively correlated with enhanced pain medication as measured by the General Health Questionnaire and the Symptom Check List (see Table 2-7). Thus, it appears that a certain subgroup of individuals with less psychological differentiation will experience increased anxiety and depression in a preoperative setting and thus will need more pain medication. The combination of a cognitive style which can augment or diminish dysphoric affects by psychological defenses directly effects pain tolerance. Specifically, individuals who are more psychologically differentiated may be able to utilize isolation and intellectualization to diminish their anxiety. Following a surgical procedure, they may be able to better focus upon aspects of their existence than their immediate global discomfort.

Table 2-7
Correlation between Preoperative Affective Status and Postoperative Medication

Postoperative Affects	N	Pain Medication	Pain Perception
Anxiety			
M + W	33	.4520**	.2635
M	11	.3498	.2267
W	22	.4406	.1319
Depression			
M + W	33	.4520**	.2635
M	11	.0000	−.0706
W	22	.1869	−.1629
SOM			
M + W	33	.3550*	.3961*
M	11	.1785	.2707
W	22	.3090	.3240
GSI			
M + W	33	.3185	.2628
M	11	.1140	.0822
W	22	.3372	.2417

*$p < .05$
**$p < .01$

Although patients with gallbladder disease experience discomfort prior to surgery, they rarely have chronic pain. Patients who undergo surgery for back pain generally have histories of chronic musculoskeletal pain. Comparison of these two groups allows a comparison of acute pain response in these two populations. The groups showed no significant difference in mean locus of control. The relationship of pain tolerance to this dimension has produced contradictory findings. This personality variable is developed from social learning theory, whereby specific expectancies and reinforcement are considered to determine behavior. Externally located individuals have a sense of fatalism, believing nothing they can do will affect their future; internally locused subjects have a sense of inner confidence of their ability to affect their fate. Auerbach ct al[22] found that an individual's specific expectations determined his adaptation to pain, not the specific locus of control. It was found that the specific preparation of an individual depended upon his internal-external style and determined his ability to tolerate noxious stimuli. Externally located individuals needed more general information, whereas internals require specific data to allay anxiety. This environmental preparation must be congruent with the individual's general coping ability. With no difference in locus of control, the two groups' disparity in emotional status and use of pain medicine reflect other factors.

The preoperative affective status of both groups did differ significantly. The group undergoing back surgery reported far more somatic complaints on the SCL-90. This dimension includes questions about both musculoskeletal as well as abdominal pain and is not weighted toward one illness. This difference is consistent with Pilowsky's observation.[23] He noted that a group of patients attending a pain clinic for primarily musculoskeletal complaints had significantly greater somatic preoccupation than a control group attending a family medical clinic. An alternative possibility is that this difference reflects the inherent dissimilarity between visceral and peripheral discomfort.[24] Most of the literature on chronic pain refers to musculoskeletal pain syndromes. These data are more applicable to the patients with back pain than those who have the visceral nausea and discomfort caused by gallbladder disease.

The significantly elevated levels of depression in the back pain group support previous observations that individuals with pain complaints from an organic basis have significant signs of depression.[25] This dysphoria may be a reaction to chronic pain, but also may reflect the generally guarded outlook of back surgery, as discomfort and disability can persist following surgery. The elevated symptom intensity level also characterizes this group, as compared to the group with gallbladder disease. Chronicity did not appear to be a factor in this difference, as both groups suffered from chronic complaints.

Thus, patients with back pain were more depressed. They reported more intense levels of global symptomatology than their cholecystectomy counterparts. The similar levels of anxiety in both groups reflect preoperative reactions to the impending surgical procedure. This similarity in both groups reflects similar styles of coping to the stress of surgery itself, not to the chronic discomfort or pain levels experienced in both groups preoperatively.

An interesting finding is that both surgical groups estimate their pain discomfort in a similar fashion, yet patients with back pain utilize more postoperative narcotics. Explanation for this difference may reflect both psychologic and biologic factors. The increased level of depression in the group undergoing back surgery may promote utilization of narcotic medication for an antidepressant effect. Excess narcotic medication has been described in individuals with chronic back pain problems.[26] This study, however, evaluated the acute pain response in individuals with chronic discomfort. All of the individuals with back pain had utilized narcotics in the past to ease their pain, whereas the patients undergoing cholecystectomy had not. This finding might reflect lowered enkephalin levels in the acute pain phenomenon in individuals who have suffered from chronic pain of musculoskeletal origin. The group with gallbladder disease had not suffered from chronic musculoskeletal pain but had suffered frequently from nausea, flatulence, and discomfort which may not be biologically similar to the chronic back pain. Almay et al[27] found that individuals with organic pain had relatively lower endorphin levels than those with psychogenic pain. The low level of endogenous opiates might account for an increased need of narcotic medication postoperatively.

In conclusion, previous investigators have utilized heterogeneous surgical populations to study postoperative pain response. This present report demonstrates that surgical populations differ in their acute pain response according to their pathologic condition, despite similar levels of pain discomfort and similar personality style. The exact reasons for this are unknown but suggest that patients with chronic pain may differ from those without chronic pain in their postoperative response to acute pain. These findings suggest that future studies of postoperative pain behavior should utilize homogeneous surgical populations.

REFERENCES

1. Mersky H: The status of pain, in Hill OW (ed): *Modern Trends in Psychosomatic Medicine.* London, Butterworths & Co, 1976, vol 3, pp 166–186.
2. Beecher HK: *Measurement of Subjective Responses.* New York, Oxford University Press, 1959.
3. Egbert LD, Battit GE, Welch CE, et al: Reduction of postoperative pain by encouragement and instruction of patients. *N Engl J Med,* 1964; 270:825–831.

4. Chapman CR, Feather BW: Effects of diazepam on human pain tolerance and pain sensitivity. *Psychosom Med* 1973;4:330–340.
5. Goldberg, DP: *The Detection of Psychiatric Illness by Questionnaire.* Maudsley Monographs, no 21. New York, Oxford University Press, 1972.
6. Derogatis LR, Rickels K, Uhlenruth EH, et al: The Hopkins Symptom Checklist (HSCL), in Pichot P, Oliver-Martin R (eds): *Psychological Measurements in Psychopharmacology*. Basel, Karger, 1974, vol 7, pp 79–110.
7. Witkin HA: Individual differences in test of perceptional embedded figures. *J Pers* 1950;19:1–15.
8. Rotter JB: Generalized expectancies for internal versus external control of reinforcement. *Psychol Monographs* 1966;80:1–28.
9. Huskisson EC: Measurement of pain. *Lancet* 1974;2:1127–1131.
10. Witkin HA: *Psychological Differentiation.* New York, John Wiley, 1962.
11. Feighner JP, Robins E, Guze SB, et al: Diagnostic criteria for use in psychiatric research. *Arch Gen Psychiatry* 1972;26:51–63.
12. Wise TN, Hall WA, Wong O: The relationship of cognitive styles and affective status to postoperative analgesic utilization. *J Psychosom Res,* to be published.
13. Graffenreid BV, Adler R, Abt K, et al: The influence of anxiety and pain sensitivity on experimental pain in man. *Pain* 1978;4:253–263.
14. Davidson PO, Neufield RWJ: Response to pain and stress: A multivariate analysis. *J Psychosom Res* 1974;18:25–32.
15. Stauffer RN: Approach to failure of lumbar spinal operations, in Ruge D, Wittse LL (eds): *Spinal Disorders.* Philadelphia, Lea and Febiger, 1977, pp 328–331.
16. Schein CJ: *Postcholecystectomy Syndromes.* Hagerstown, Harper and Row Publishers Inc, 1978.
17. Wise TN: Pain—the most common psychosomatic problem. *Med Clin North Am* 1977;61:771–780.
18. Sweeney DR, Fine BH: Pain reactively and field dependence. *Percept Mot Skills* 1965;21:757–758.
19. Johnson JE, Leventhal H, Dabbs JM: Contribution of emotional and instrumental response processes in adaptation to surgery. *J Pers Soc Psych* 1971;20:55–64.
20. Adler R, Lemassy F: Perceptual style and pain tolerance I. The influence of certain psychological factors. *J Psychosom Res* 1973;17:369–379.
21. Karp S: Psychological differentiation, in Thomas B (ed): *Personality Variables in Social Behavior.* Hillsdale, NJ, Halsted Press, 1977, vol 12, p 44.
22. Auerbach SM, Kendall PC, Cuttler HF, et al: Anxiety, locus of control, type of preparatory information and adjustment to dental surgery. *J Consult Clin Psychol* 1976;44:809–818.
23. Pilowsky I: The diagnosis of abnormal illness behavior. *Aust NZ J Psychiatry* 1971;5:136–138.
24. Chapman WP, Jones CM: Variations in cutaneous and visceral pain sensitivity in normal subjects. *J Clin Invest* 1944;23:81–91.
25. Mersky H, Boyd D: Emotional adjustment and chronic pain. *Pain* 1978;5:173–178.
26. Halpern LM: Psychotropic drugs in the management of chronic pain. *Adv Neurol* 1974;539–545..
27. Almay BGL, Johansson F, Knorring LV, et al: Endorphins in chronic pain. I. *Pain* 1978;5:153–162.

3 Placebo Effects on Pain: Medical History and Medical Reasoning about Pain

Jacques M. Quen

In 1683, Willem Ten Rhijne, a Dutch physician, published the first detailed report of acupuncture in Western medical literature. In 1774, Franz Anton Mesmer observed that patients improved when he treated them with magnets. In 1795, Elisha Perkins, a Connecticut physician, discovered that he could treat painful conditions by stroking the affected parts with a simple knife blade. These three methods of treatment had several traits in common. Each was foreign to traditional Western medicine as derived from Arabic and Graeco-Roman medicine. Furthermore, each was rejected by the medical profession with labels such as charlatanry, fraud, and humbug. They also shared a remarkable effectiveness for patients who had not responded favorably to conventional medical treatments of their time.

The histories of these three methods of treatment and receptions by their medical communities provide a perspective on persistent vulnerabilities of medical reasoning, especially when applied to

This study was supported in part by NIMH Grant #3-RO3-MH23967-01S1 therapeutic phenomena which are explained by fallacious or inadequate theories.

Mesmerism

Franz Anton Mesmer, an Austrian physician intrigued by the conviction that planetary forces influenced human physiology, used magnets in his treatment of patients. He soon realized that he could dispense with the physical magnets and use his personality and body to focus and direct the "animal magnetism." He conceived of this as a force separate and distinct from physical or mineral magnetism. Mesmer postulated that the magnetism was transmitted by a universal ether or ethereal fluid which was invisible but responsive to the powers of the magnetizer or operator. Mesmer's treatment of a blind young woman, and his claims of cure, led to controversy and to his eventual departure from Austria. He went to Paris in 1778 and soon became sought after for his treatment. The notoriety generated by Mesmer and his methods resulted in the appointment of a royal commission, chaired nominally, by the American ambassador, Benjamin Franklin. Franklin appears to have played almost no role in the investigation or the writing of the report. The commission's report was published in 1784. It exposed Mesmer's theory of the physical basis of his method as fallacious and attributed its effectiveness to the patient's "imagination." The bulk of the French medical community rejected Mesmerism while a small group of physicians retained interest in it. In 1829, M Jules Cloquet, a reputable surgeon, reported a painless mastectomy done on a lady under mesmeric anesthesia.

In 1837 the French Baron duPotet came to England to demonstrate the medical value of Mesmerism. He met John Elliotson, Professor of the Practice of Medicine at the University of London College of Medicine, who became interested in it. Elliotson gained much notoriety from his use of Mesmerism and soon became its British champion. In 1843 he published a small pamphlet on the surgical use of mesmeric anesthesia, including a report of a leg amputation, during which the mesmerized patient showed no sign of pain. Elliotson described the medical society meeting at which the case was reported; accusations of fraud committed by the patient, if not the surgeon as well, were made by various physicians in the audience.

James Esdaile, a British surgeon in India, independently reported his series of various surgical procedures under mesmeric anesthesia in 1845. Once again, accusations of fraud arose, this time aimed at the Indian patients who were "fooling" the surgeons by intentionally refusing to manifest signs of pain! At about this time, an American physician at the Medical College of Georgia published a report of his performance of a painless mastectomy under mesmeric anesthesia. The following month, a fellow surgeon on the faculty published a lecture in which he maintained that Mesmerism "is not a reality . . . the phenomena ascribed to it are firstly due to the imagination and excited feelings . . . [furthermore] non-expression of pain is not proof of its non-existence."

It was in this same period that nitrous oxide and ether anesthesia made their appearance. One can almost hear the note of triumphant relief in the voice of Robert Liston, British surgeon and adamant opponent of mesmeric anesthesia, as he said, "This Yankee dodge beats Mesmerism hollow." However, it should be recognized that mesmeric (hypnotic) anesthesia remains the one with the least morbidity and least mortality of any other surgical anesthetic (except, possibly, acupuncture anesthesia).

Perkinism

In 1795, Elisha Perkins, a founder of the Connecticut State Medical Society and president of his county medical society, discovered that by stroking painful areas of the human body with a simple knife blade, he could induce the relief of pain as well as facilitate healing. He wrote to several physician friends describing his method and urged them to try it for themselves. In 1796, he obtained what was probably the first patent for a medical device issued in the United States. It was for a pair of metallic rods of elongated tear drop shape, one gold in color and one silver in color. He maintained that these Tractors, as he called them, when stroked alternately over the diseased part, would draw out the excess "Electroid" fluid and provide relief and cure. He died in 1799 when he journeyed to New York, then in the midst of a virulent yellow fever epidemic, in order to try a treatment method utilizing his Tractors.

His son, Benjamin, not a physician, had been sent by Perkins to England somewhat earlier to introduce the Tractors there. The treatment method was welcomed enthusiastically by some and rejected by others. In 1801, John Haygarth, a brilliant physician at Bath, reported several experiments in which fake Tractors, made of bone, wood, and wax, as well as genuine ones were used. There was remarkable functional improvement in almost all cases treated. The exceptions were those patients who experienced painful side effects during or after treatment.

Benjamin, with the support of many prominent Englishmen, founded the Perkinean Society to treat the poor with these Tractors. By 1804, Benjamin Perkins, now a Quaker, left England with £10 thousand, the equivalent in today's money of about $100,000.

By 1811, the Tractors seem to have been forgotten except as an example of rank quackery. They were immortalized in Byron's *English Bards and Scotch Reviewers:*

What varied wonders tempt us as they pass!
The Cow-pox, Tractors, Galvanism, Gas,
In turns appear to make the vulgar stare,
Till the swoll'n bubble bursts—and all is air.

Byron was referring to the then new chemical experiments isolating gases, to early experiments with electricity, and, of course, to vaccination. Of the four, it appears that only the Tractors turned out to be "air." Here too, however, we may find that the Tractors were a premature demonstration of an unappreciated biological capability.

In 1970, two historians of psychiatry at the Payne Whitney Clinic, New York Hospital-Cornell Medical Center, published a study of Mesmerism and Perkinism. They observed that the Franklin Commission was "not interested in the possible use of animal magnetism and dismissed the fact that it did produce effects, along with their dismissal of the specious theory on which it rested." Carlson and Simpson concluded their study with the provocative reflection that "Mesmer's elegant clinic with its impressive paraphernalia and Perkins's simple if expensive Tractors were dismissed equally by the majority of the men of science. Mesmer and Perkins had drawn in similar fashion on popular theories of physics of their day in order to explain their therapeutic successes, but once the true sources of their cures, imagination and suggestion became apparent, the whole matter was pushed aside. The powers of suggestion had been dramatically demonstrated, but for legitimate medicine there seemed no way to put this curious weapon to use."

Acupuncture

In 1810, a French physician, LVJ Berlioz, treated a 24-year-old woman suffering from "nervous fever and gastralgia" with common sewing needles inserted directly into the area of pain for varying periods of time. The following year he reported his experiences to the Paris Academy of Medicine and in 1816 published a report of his needle technique for the successful treatment of whooping cough, contusions, headaches, and severe muscle aches and pains. He suggested that asphyxiated individuals for whom conventional medical measures had failed might be revived by puncturing the right ventricle and passing a galvanic current through the needle.

By 1826 there were reports of successful treatment of neuralgias (including sciatica and tic douloureux), acute and chronic rheumatism, trismus, pleurodynia, asthma, gout, ophthalmia, pleurisy, enteritis, orchitis, and intractable hiccups.

In England, James Morss Churchill, published two books and one article describing his encouraging experiences with acupuncture as a treatment method between 1821 and 1828. In 1828, John Elliotson reported a three-year study of 42 consecutive cases of rheumatism treated with acupuncture at St. Thomas's Hospital. Thirty patients were improved or cured, while the other 12, with acutely inflamed and hot joints, showed no improvement. Elliotson concluded that acupuncture was definitely indicated and effective for chronic rheumatism. English physicians also experimented with the use of galvano-puncture for the treatment of paralyzed muscles and found it quite successful in restoring function. One might well conclude that the basis for the technology and the idea for electromyography was the experimental work of the early English acupuncturists.

Western physicians believed their acupuncture technique was based upon the oriental method. In fact, there is no evidence of any understanding of the oriental concepts of *yin* and *yang* energies, of the oriental understanding of human anatomy, or of the use of oriental acupuncture charts (although these had been referred to and illustrated in the early Western literature on acupuncture). Western physicians, beginning with Berlioz, would insert the needle directly over and deeply into the painful area. The usual response was the amelioration or disappearance of the pain within several minutes. Occasionally, the pain would migrate and the physician would pursue it with a needle insertion at the new site. This might require several punctures, but eventually the pain, if it would respond at all, would leave. The striking thing about these results is that patients were reported to be asymptomatic for weeks, months, or permanently.

Insertion of the needle was often painless, while removal would cause pain. This was a result of oxidation, and consequent roughening, of the needle surface while inserted. Acupuncturists would often place a tab of sealing wax at the eye of the needle to prevent it from accidentally working its way into the body, and to facilitate insertion with finger pressure. Western scientists were unable to construct a theory of action that was generally acceptable. Clinicians who used the techniques fairly successfully appeared to accept its effectiveness without serious concern for this lack of explanation. The medical community was to be divided into two camps, those who accepted and used acupuncture, and those who rejected it because there was no basis in Western scientific theory for an understanding of the phenomenon.

John Elliotson observed: "The modus operandi of acupuncture is unknown. It is neither fear nor confidence; since those who care nothing about being acupunctured, and those who laugh at their medical attendant for proposing such a remedy, derive the same benefit, if their case is suitable, as those who are alarmed and those who submit to it with faith. Neither is it counter-irritation; since the same benefit is experienced when not the least pain is occasioned, as when pain is felt. Galvanism likewise fails to explain; because although the needle becomes oxidated and affords galvanic phenomena while in the body, these phenomena bear no proportion to their benefit, [they] equally take place when acupuncture is practiced upon a healthy person, and do not take place when needles of gold or silver are employed, which, however, are equally efficacious with a needle of steel."

In the 1830s, John Renton, a Scottish physician acupuncturist, reflected upon the difficulty of getting the medical community to accept acupuncture. He commented, "The utility of a specific is very readily suspected, when its infallibility is given out for the removal of too many diseases, and more particularly of those between which no analogy can be traced. And when, moreover, no satisfactory explanation can be afforded of the *modus operandi* of the reagent, professional persons, unhappily for the interests of medical science, are too apt to reason upon the authenticity of the facts averred, instead of adopting the more simple and direct method of determining their value by subjecting them to the fact of further experience."

The Leeds Infirmary in England used acupuncture in its treatment of musculoskeletal disorders through, at least, 1871, when a report of their experience was published in *Lancet.* As late as 1879, the French physician, Dumontpallier at La Pitié, experimented with variations of acupuncture and found that inserting the needle at the contralateral site of pain was effective. While this was the first instance of insertion of the needle at an anatomically distant site from the apparent lesion, no reference was made to the Chinese system and its charts for "indirect" acupuncture.

In 1892, William Osler, in his classic *Principles and Practice of Medicine,* recommended direct acupuncture into the site of pain as an excellent specific treatment for lumbago. "For lumbago, acupuncture is, in acute cases, the most efficient treatment. Needles of from three to four inches in length (ordinary bonnet needles, sterilized, will do) are thrust into the lumbar muscles at the seat of the pain, and withdrawn after five or ten minutes. In many instances the relief is immediate, and I can corroborate fully the statements of [Sidney] Ringer [the British physician physiologist], who taught me this practice, as to its extraordinary and prompt efficacy in many instances." Osler also recommended acupuncture for the treatment of sciatica. He continued to recommend acupuncture through the tenth edition of his book.

In 1971, four American physicians visited the People's Republic of China. They returned with a favorable view of much of medical education and practice there. They were, perhaps, most impressed by what they saw of the use of acupuncture for surgical anesthesia. Samuel Rosen, the noted ear surgeon of Mount Sinai Hospital (NY), reported, "When you see these operations, you come out and you pinch yourself.

You wonder if you really saw what you saw. After you have seen it over and over, you have to give up what you thought in favor of what you saw."

For medical historians, there was a déjà vu quality to the receptions the public and the medical community gave to these reports. One former Congressman and a former medical missionary to China asserted, "The communists are feeding us a lot of baloney. Our people on the specially guided tours that Peking has set up for them have been brain-washed and don't know it; the tour guides are pure propagandists." Another physician, after reading the reports, decided that acupuncture anesthesia was merely "hypnotism in slow motion." Yet another suggested a histamine response as the underlying mechanism. Still another, with no apparent experience with acupuncture technique, theory, or history, pronounced, "Neither the diagnostic nor therapeutic technique has any basis." Lewis Thomas, president of the Memorial Sloan-Kettering Cancer Center said, "These are bad times for reason, all around. Suddenly all of the major ills are being coped with by acupuncture . . ." With all of this going on, the scientific and questioning attitude of cardiologist Paul Dudley White called for increased respect. "If it were the world's best technique we'd all be using it. If it were useless it would have been dropped thousands of years ago. There's something in it, but it's difficult to say just what."

Discussion

These three "quack" methods were rejected and condemned by the bulk of the physicians of their periods. They stand as a collective monument to the prejudices and complacency of physicians who speak of adherence to the scientific method without understanding it. Despite the reports of painless surgery, there was refusal to be curious beyond an immediate rejection of the possibility of the reality of the phenomenon. For them, it was sufficient to say, as one eminent physician did, "It is unphysiological." One American surgeon, unwilling to publicly accuse his colleague of gross fraud, cautioned his students not to be misled by a patient's nonexpression of pain. Remember, he told them, that the nonexpression of pain is not proof of its nonexistence. He was unable to see how curiously wonderful was the nonexpression of pain in a procedure that inherently and "physiologically" was excruciatingly painful. He was unable, apparently, to wonder how people could be induced to do this, or to wonder how it could be applied in the service of improving medical care.

Professor Eve was not alone. It is even more difficult to understand the narrow intellectual complacency of the Franklin Commission in its decision not to investigate the clinical phenomena of Mesmerism once the fallacy of Mesmer's theory and the involvement of the imagination had been demonstrated. It is particularly striking in view of Franklin's previous position on the utility and the puzzle of the mechanism of his own discovery, the lightning rod. "It is of real use to know that China [dishware] left in the air unsupported will fall and break; but how it comes to fall, and why it breaks, are matters of speculation. It is a pleasure indeed to know them, but we can preserve our China without it. Thus . . . to know this power of [lightning rods] may . . . be of use to mankind, though we should never be able to explain it." (At that time, electricity was postulated to be a nonsubstantial fluid with unique properties.)

How much more admirable was the attitude expressed by Benjamin Rush in a lecture to medical students in 1789. "I reject the futile pretensions of Mr. Mesmer to the cure of diseases, by what he has absurdly called animal magnetism. But I am willing to derive the same advantages from his deceptions, which the chemists have derived from the delusions of the alchemists. The facts which he has established, clearly prove the influence of the imagination, and the will, upon diseases. Let us avail ourselves of the handle which those faculties of the mind present to us in the strife between life and death."

The persistent coexistence of medical interest in and medical rejection of hypnotism is a curious fact. How can medicine account for it? Despite the apparent potential usefulness of hypnotic phenomena in the service of clinical care, it has been kept on the periphery of respectable medicine and is only infrequently taught in medical schools or hospitals. One might add that it is equally striking that we are no closer to an understanding of the *how* and *what* of hypnotism than we were when we called it Mesmerism.

Perkins's Tractors are an equally enigmatic puzzle in the history of the medical treatment of pain. That they did not work in the way postulated by their inventor is uncontestable. That treatment with them allowed chronically disabled patients, for whom conventional medicine had failed, to return to a remarkably increased level of function is equally uncontestable. In fact, it was the detractors of the treatment who demonstrated so forcefully the degree to which the belief in the Tractors could provide major and persistent improvement.

It is particularly striking that the opening paragraph of Haygarth's report says, "That faculty of the mind which is denominated the Imagination . . . has not wholly escaped the notice of medical writers but merits their further investigation. This slight Essay may, perhaps incite others to prosecute the inquiry more fully, in order to extend the power of physicians to prevent and cure the maladies of mankind." Despite this apparent attitude, the body of the report communicates a disparagement of those who believe that the observed improvements are based on a real therapeutic effect, rather than realizing it is merely the working of the imagination.

It is ironic that Haygarth dedicated his publication to his friend, William Falconer, who had helped and advised in the design of Haygarth's experiment. It was Falconer who had the honor, in 1786, of winning the first Fothergillian Medal, offered by the London Medical Society, for the dissertation that best answered the question "What diseases may be mitigated or cured, by exciting particular affections or passions of the mind?" Despite Falconer's concern with the use of the mind in the treatment of disease, his friend, Haygarth, was unable to conceive of it as a respectable weapon in the medical armamentarium, nor as a curiously valid aspect of Perkinism.

While nineteenth-century acupuncture was not the target of vehement attacks, nevertheless, it was largely rejected as a nonspecific mode of treatment that had no scientific basis. In the latter half of the twentieth century, as in the nineteenth, physicians with minimal experience or study of the process have been quick to "shoot from the hip" and label it, eg, hypnotism in slow motion, histamine effect, suggestion, or fraud, rather than withhold judgment, postpone closure on the question, and wait for the results of sober and careful reflection and study. Unfortunately, even the more temperate and sophisticated contemporary investigators have tended to adopt controls based on the classical Chinese acupuncture charts without recognizing that these do not serve as controls for the efficacy of needle punctures as a therapeutic mode, but rather controls for the validity and reliability of the Chinese theory.

Invocation of the "imagination" in the nineteenth century and of the "placebo effect" in the twentieth century have, unfortunately for medicine, given rise to confusion between labeling and understanding. Nor has such practice allowed physicians to cultivate curiosity about the mechanism of imagination or of the placebo effect in alleviating disability. While one would like to be hopeful that the recent work suggesting a real, ie, organic and demonstrable, connection between acupuncture and endorphin/enkephalin activity in the brain will lead to a more receptive and respected curiosity about the mode of action of psychological factors in human disability in the organic sphere, it is not likely.

What factors other than objective performance criteria enter into the evaluation of a proposed treatment method? What determines which therapeutic modes a medical community or a society will accept? It appears that as long as we are aware of anatomical or chemical aspects to the relief of pain, professional medicine is willing to accept the reality of that symptom relief. We could not accept the reality of mesmeric anesthesia, but we had almost no problem in accepting the reality of chemical anesthesia. We had no problem accepting pain relief through transcutaneous electrical stimulation, chordotomy, or "gate theories," but we could not accept surgical acupuncture anesthesia.

It is striking that as one looks at our chronic pain clinics one is accepting a mode of treating pain which says we accept that we can do nothing to relieve the chronic pain directly, but we can relieve and change your attitude to it by creating an environment which nearly forces you to reorder your values and your perception of pain so that you can function better. Yet, how is this different from what Haygarth concluded was being done with Perkins's Tractors? What accounts for the fact that as a profession we have rejected the one and accepted the other? And what has stopped us from recognizing that such terms as "imagination" and "placebo effect" are obscuring labels for real phenomena? And what stops us from recognizing that, as a profession, we are obliged to try to understand better the mode of action of the mind in these instances in order to better serve our patients?

BIBLIOGRAPHY

Carlson ET, Simpson MM: Perkinism vs. Mesmerism. *J Hist Behav Sci* 1970;6:16–24.

Dimond EG: Medical education and care in People's Republic of China. *JAMA* 1971;218:1552–1557.

Dimond EG: Acupuncture anesthesia: Western medicine and Chinese traditional medicine. *JAMA* 1971;218:1558–1563.

Falconer W: *A Dissertation on the Influence of the Passions Upon Disorders of the Body.* London, C Dilly and J Phillips, 1788.

Haygarth J: *Of the Imagination as a Cause and as a Cure of Disorders of the Body.* Bath, R Cruttwell, 1800.

Podmore F: *From Mesmer to Christian Science: A Short History of Mental Healing.* London, GW Jacobs, 1909.

Quen JM: Elisha Perkins, physician, nostrum-vendor, or charlatan? *Bull Hist Med* 1963;37:159–166.

Quen JM: Case studies in nineteenth century scientific rejection: Mesmerism, Perkinism, and acupuncture. *J Hist Behav Sci* 1975;11:149–156.

Quen JM: Acupuncture and Western medicine. *Bull Hist Med* 1975;49:196–205.

Quen JM: Mesmerism, medicine, and professional prejudice. *NY State J Med* 1976;76:2218–2222.

SECTION II
Diagnosis and Clinical Tests

4 The Evaluation and Treatment of Low Back Pain

Donlin M. Long

Low back pain is one of the most common complaints for which patients seek the attention of a physician. Nonmedical surveys indicate that it may be an important problem for at least 25% of the population of the United States. Acute and chronic low back pain together represent one of the most common reasons for hospitalization. Furthermore, unsuccessfully treated low back pain represents the single most common cause of an intractable disabling pain syndrome. Nevertheless, the syndrome is quite straightforward and can be satisfactorily treated most of the time. The key is a proper diagnosis and institution of the measures which will relieve symptoms in most patients. The problems stem from lack of an adequate diagnosis, failure to recognize participating psychologic and sociologic causes, and the application of improper treatments because of the failure of diagnosis. Serious failures are also precipitated by patients who refuse to follow a conservative program which would provide satisfactory pain relief and by patients who refuse to accept that psychologic factors may be important in their pain.

The Evaluation of the Complaint of Low Back Pain

As with any disease state, the evaluation begins with a complete history and general physical examination. The history is very important. It is first important to determine the location and the character of the pain. Pain which is in the back only likely arises from degenerative disc disease, instability, or muscle spasm. It is also possible that some local manifestation of systemic disease is present. If the pain is worsened by activity and improved by rest, then its mechanical nature is almost certain. If the leg pain is not radicular in character but radiates into the hip or in a nondescript fashion down the leg, it is important to determine hip movement is related to the pain and to be certain that hip disease is not an important part of the problem. Truly radicular pain is usually easy to identify. The pain radiates down the course of the sciatic nerve according to which root is involved. Compression of the S-1 root gives pain which radiates to the heel and lateral side of the foot. Compression of the L-5 root gives pain which goes to the lateral side of the leg and over the dorsum of the foot toward the great toe. Compression of the L-4 root causes pain in the back of the leg and on the medial side of the calf. The clear-cut sciatic nature of the pain makes nerve root compression easy to identify. The history will also be helpful in differentiating vascular disease and spinal stenosis. Both are characterized by a history of exercise intolerance, with pain and weakness being brought on by exercise. However, the back pain and leg pain of vascular disease is almost always associated with typical physical signs of vascular insufficiency, whereas the same symptoms precipitated by spinal stenosis are seen in the presence of a normal vascular examination.

The physical examination is quite straightforward and does not require anything very profound in the way of a neurological examination. Of course, a general examination should be carried out though there are not a great many systemic diseases that present with back pain. Among these are diabetes mellitus, metastatic cancer, paravertebral abscess, and retroperitoneal disease such as aortic aneurysm. Hip disease may masquerade as a chronic back problem and the hip should be examined carefully.

The examination of the low back begins with inspection. The back is carefully assessed for the presence or absence of muscle spasm and curvature. Range of motion of the back and hips are tested. Looking for compression and percussion over the spine and areas of tenderness is worthwhile. Stretch reflexes are tested. A diminished knee reflex is suggestive of 4th root compression. A diminished ankle reflex is suggestive of S-1 root compression, and a diminished posterior tibial reflex suggests L-5 compression. Muscle strength is tested throughout. Quadriceps weakness suggests L-4 compression. Dorsiflexion of the great toe is subserved by L-5 and plantar flexion weakness suggests S-1 compression. A sensory examination by pinprick and light touch should be performed. The sole and lateral side of the foot is innervated by S-1, the area around the base of the great toe, the dorsum of the foot, and lateral side of the leg by L-5, and the medial side of the leg by L-4. The vascular sufficiency of the lower extremities should be assessed, hip movement performed, and straight leg raising carried out. A positive straight leg raising test which reproduces radicular pain is highly suggestive of root compression, and a crossed straight raising test in which lifting the opposite leg reproduces radicular pain is almost certain evidence of disc herniation.

A combination of history and physical examination will make a preliminary diagnosis accurately most of the time. The diagnosis of nerve root compression and a truly herniated intervertebral disc is generally quite straightforward. Such patients will be incapacitated by a combination of back and radicular leg pain. Straight leg raising will be acutely positive producing radicular sciatic pain and mimicking the patient's pain state. If the disc fragment is completely herniated, straight leg raising will usually be crossed as well. A diminished knee reflex, weakness of the quadriceps, and sensory loss on the medial side of the leg suggests L-4 root compression. A diminished posterior tibial reflex, weakness of dorsiflexion of the foot and toes, and sensory loss on the lateral side of the leg, dorsum of the foot, and base of the great toe suggests L-5 root compression. Absence of the Achilles reflex, weakness of plantar flexion, and sensory loss on the sole and lateral side of the foot are indicative of S-1 root compression. Disc herniations at higher levels are very rare. When the pain is located in the back only or is associated with nonradicular radiation, it is unlikely that a truly herniated intervertebral disc is present and the underlying problem is much more likely to be myofascial or simply secondary to degenerative disc disease.

Laboratory Examinations

In an acute situation, when there is no evidence of significant neurological loss, it is unlikely that even x-ray films are necessary. If the pain relents promptly with conservative care, there is no need to go further in the evaluation. However, in most instances plain roentgenograms are valuable. These should include anterior, posterior, and lateral views of the lumbar spine, oblique views to demonstrate the facets, and flexion-extension films. These films will demonstrate disc degeneration, abnormal movement, osteoarthritic changes, particularly around the facets, and will also serve to eliminate the possibility of another unusual problem such as metastatic cancer, Paget's disease, or an unusual disease of the discs. In the initial phases of evaluation, other studies are not necessary. However, there are some circumstances in which additional studies will be useful. Electromyography can be utilized to determine minor degrees of root injury when no physical findings are present. Electromyographic abnormalities will help in deciding whether a myelogram is indicated or not in a patient who has less than classic findings and who fails to improve with conservative therapy. Thermography is utilized for the same purpose and will demonstrate minimal degrees of sensory and autonomic abnormality of a radicular character. Screening tests for rheumatoid arthritis are often valuable but need not be routine, and a fasting blood sugar should be done in recalcitrant cases that do not respond to general conservative care.

The major decision which always must be made is whether or not a myelogram or other interventional diagnostic studies should be done. This is a clinical decision and will be elaborated upon later. However, the definitive test for disc herniation is myelography. The myelogram serves only to distinguish the herniated intervertebral disc and assures that there is no other interspinal pathology. It should be used carefully for clear-cut clinical indications. It is not a screening test and there is no reason to perform it unless the clinical indications for potential surgical therapy are present. Standard myelography is carried out by a radiopaque oil. Water soluble dyes are now available and have real merit since the dye does not have to be removed and residual dye will, therefore, not be a problem.

There are other tests which have been suggested to be useful in disc diagnosis. Epidural venography has been employed instead of myelography. Comparative studies are not yet available to determine if the technique is as reliable as the less complicated and well-studied myelogram. Radioactive bone scan may occasionally be of value, but is primarily useful when disc space infection is suspected or when sacroiliac joint disease is present. Occult metastases may also be demonstrated on a bone scan. Discography has been advocated by some. Its interpretation has been perfected by a small number of surgeons who are highly skilled in its use. However, discography has never enjoyed the universal popularity of the myelogram. Like the myelogram, the discogram is a surgical tool. It is rarely used in straightforward diagnosis but is a part of the surgical management program.

Conservative Management of the Low Back Pain

Unless the patient has a progressive or serious neurological deficit, it is unlikely that any operative therapy will be indicated until after a thorough trial of what is termed "conservative care." Conservative programs will be very helpful for the majority of patients with chronic lumbar complaints and should be employed before any operative intervention is contemplated. In general, there is no need to carry out a myelogram or discogram until the trial of conservative care has been utilized. These tests are to guide surgical decision making and are not necessary for diagnosis, since the therapy of all of the chronic back conditions is approximately the same. Once the history, physical examination, and noninterventional ancillary studies are complete, a conservative program for solving the patient's pain problem can be outlined. If the pain is severe and the patient seriously incapacitated, it is usually best to begin with bedrest. This can be carried out at home, but if compliance at home is a problem for the patient, it is wiser to hospitalize the patient. The bedrest should be as strict as possible. Drug therapy for a short period of time may be useful. Analgesics up to and including codeine are useful. Injectable narcotics virtually are never indicated in this phase of therapy. Severe muscle spasm can be treated with muscle relaxants. The most commonly used are carisoprodol and methocarbamol. Diazepam can be utilized for a short period of time, usually no more than one to two weeks. If aspirin is used as the analgesic, then no other anti-inflammatory medication is required. When aspirin is not utilized, then an anti-inflammatory agent such as ibuprofen, 400 mg 3 or 4 times a day, can be utilized. Most patients tolerate these long periods of bed rest in the hospital poorly and, if at all possible, bed rest at home is desirable.

If the muscle spasm is severe, then physical therapy techniques may be useful in providing rapid symptomatic relief. Massage and heat are useful adjuncts with bed rest and other physical modalities such as ultrasound, ice packs, and whirlpool may be useful. However, there is little information that these active physical therapy techniques are of great value in changing the initial phase of the acute low back syndrome. Unless there is a specific problem to treat, such as severe muscle spasm, it is probable that bedrest alone will be as successful.

One of the greatest advances in the management of these kinds of problems has been the advent of transcutaneous electrical stimulation. The technique is now gaining wide acceptance in physical therapy circles. The use of transcutaneous electrical stimulation in the acute phase of the low back syndrome will provide prompt relief of muscle spasm, rapid control of pain, and it appears will greatly accelerate the patient's recovery. There have been no definitive studies to prove these points in well-controlled situations, but the patients treated by most of the individuals who have utilized transcutaneous stimulation in the treatment of chronic pain have demonstrated rapid symptomatic relief. The electrodes are simply placed in the lumbar area in painful regions, particularly over the paravertebral muscles, and pain relief is usually quite satisfactory, occurring within a few minutes of application. Patients are allowed to use the devices at home following adequate education, and most can achieve satisfactory relief within a several week period.

In the event that the symptoms are not relieved with two to four weeks of this therapy, it may be necessary to hospitalize the patient for more definitive physical therapy. This is usually done after a minimum trial of at least two weeks of the simple conservative measures. Then, in-patient physical therapy, strict bed rest, and the use of lumbar traction are all indicated. In addition, the situation should be reassessed to be certain that the underlying diagnosis is correct. In the absence of clear cut radicular signs and symptoms, there is no indication for myelography or for consideration of an operative procedure. During this period of time, any patient who has failed to achieve good relief with straightforward conservative measures should be carefully evaluated from a psychological standpoint, to be certain that there are no underlying psychological factors which may be important in the continued complaint of pain. Personal problems, work-related factors, and a prior history suggesting personality disorder are all important in potentially magnifying a minor pain syndrome and incapacitating the patient beyond the degree which would be expected by the physical nature of the pain state. In the absence of these factors, the usual acute back syndrome responds promptly to conservative care.

At the termination of the hospitalization, it is well to consider back immobilization through a brace. However, it must be recognized that the brace is a temporary technique designed to protect the back from further injury and is not a therapeutic end in itself. Braces should be used with an adequate exercise program to strengthen the low back. The second subacute phase of therapy consists of weight control if the patient is overweight, the use of nonnarcotics analgesics, muscle relaxants, and the strict avoidance of narcotics, assessment of all psychological factors and attention to those which may be important, continued use of physical therapy modalities, transcutaneous stimulation, and an adequate exercise program and bracing. Patients should be urged to return to work whenever possible and the total time off from work and the disability should be minimized except where the physical abnormalities are obvious.

The exercises employed are the William's flexion exercises. Many variations of these techniques are available but should improve strength in abdominal and paravertebral muscles and increased mobility of the low back, hips, thighs, and knees. Therefore, the exercises should both strengthen and stretch. It probably does not make much difference which of these exercise programs is used as long as these basic principles are kept in mind.

The Management of the Acutely Herniated Lumbar Disc

The therapy used for the acutely herniated lumbar disc is very similar to that used for the patient who does not harbor a disc herniation and has only suffered a musculoskeletal injury to the back. The patient with a true disc herniation will virtually always have a radicular complaint. Nevertheless, unless there is a rapidly progressing neurological loss or a serious neurological deficit, conservative care is still the preferred therapy. The treatment should be identical to that already listed, except that the patient is more likely to require early hospitalization because of the severity of the radicular pain. If the patient fails to improve at all with one to two weeks of bedrest and radicular symptoms continue, then myelography is indicated. If the patient is improving, even in the face of a minor neurological deficit, then conservative care should continue. In the event that improvement does not occur, a lumbar myelogram should be carried out. It should be stressed that the lumbar myelogram should always visualize the lower end of the spinal cord to be certain that no occult lesion is located in this area. In the event that a truly herniated intervertebral disc is seen, then lumbar surgery is indicated. The results of surgery for real herniated discs are excellent with over 90% of patients being permanently relieved of their symptoms. Lumbar surgery for any other condition which might be found is considerably less satisfactory, and early surgery should be contemplated only in the presence of a truly herniated disc. Specifically, surgery for the degenerated disc is not likely to achieve satisfactory results and should be avoided unless clear-cut radicular signs and nerve root compression are present.

The Management of the Chronic Low Back Syndrome

A small percentage of patients will continue to complain of low back pain in spite of completely satisfactory management. These patients should always be thoroughly reevaluated to be certain of the etiology of the pain. This will include repeat of the roentgenograms, careful review of preexisting studies, and repeat myelography if they are not entirely satisfactory or if they are suspicious, and careful reassessment of psychological factors to determine if important psychosocial events have been overlooked. In addition to review of the standard programs, it is worthwhile looking into some specific syndromes which may be important in the continued genesis of pain. The first of these is the so-called "facet syndrome." Minor degrees of lumbar instability may be manifested as back pain. The characteristic signs will be back pain which is aggravated by activity and improved by rest. Leg pain is possible, but the pain will always be nonradicular and radiate only into the hip, groin, or in a nondescript fashion down the leg no lower than the knee. The diagnosis is verified by infiltration of the lower lumbar facets with local anesthetic. The diagnosis is important to make because a new technique, radiofrequency destruction of nerves innervating the facets, is possible. The technique is simple, straightforward, and requires only local anesthetic. Complications are extremely rare and the procedure is effective in relieving pain over 70% of the time.

The second syndrome which must be clearly identified is a more serious problem of stability. Flexion-extension films should be carefully reviewed for signs of movement. Immobilization of the back in a plaster jacket is often indicated at this point. If the pain is completely relieved, then it is likely that lumbar fusion would be satisfactory for long-term control of symptoms. However, it is also acceptable to use a carefully constructed brace or plastic jacket over a long period of time as an alternative fusion.

In the event that conservative care does not improve the situation, then myelography to be certain there is no unsuspected lesion is indicated. However, the simple fact that there is evidence of disc degeneration is not an indication for surgery. If clear-cut pathology is not demonstrated by the combination of studies, a conservative program is still the best therapy for these patients.

Evaluation and Therapy of the Chronic Low Back Cripple

There are a significant number of patients who undergo multiple ineffectual operations in the treatment of low back complaints. The reasons for this are many but, in general, relate either to an unrecognized psychiatric problem or an unexpected complication of a lumbar operation. Reconstruction of the history very often indicates that the patient did not have a radicular component to the pain syndrome. The operation was frequently done for a complaint of back pain only without the extensive conservative trial that would be indicated by this complaint. Once the patient has had more than one operation, the situation becomes different than exists in those patients who have not had multiple procedures. The cause of the pain is much more difficult to decipher. There are multiple reasons why such patients have pain. There may be an incompletely closed incision, a painful donor site, fibrosis in the paravertebral muscles, surgically induced instability, recurrent disc herniation, continued pressure upon a nerve root by scar, involvement of multiple nerve roots by epidural scarring, compression of the entire cauda equina by extradural scar, and arachnoiditis with caudal compression intradurally. The basic examination in such patients is the same, except that the physical examination should include careful attention to the condition of the wound and assessment of fusion donor sites as possible pain generators. The ancillary studies are the same, but myelography is almost mandatory to determine the exact status of the back. Stability can be assessed by the application of a body cast. Perhaps the most effective way to determine the origin of the pain is by diagnostic blocks. Trigger points in the incision or muscle can be injected. The fusion donor site can be infiltrated with local anesthetic. The innervation of the facets can be blocked, assessing stability at this level. Individual root blocks can be carried out. Localized epidural or differential spinal blocks will often determine the exact level of the lesion. Sympathetic blocks can be used to assess any autonomic component in the pain, particularly if the pain has a burning character, and the disc may be injected with local anesthetic. A combination of these blocks judiciously chosen to match the patient's complaints and physical findings will usually give a clear picture of the origin of the pain.

The treatment of the chronic low back cripple is much more complicated than the patient with a straightforward back problem. There is little evidence that reoperation is of benefit to these patients, except for very specific syndromes. Therefore, the management should be as conservative as possible. This will include all of those things utilized in managing primary back conditions, weight control, adequate bracing, and adequate exercise program, mild analgesics, and physical therapy for specific indications such as chronic muscle spasm or myositis. The long-term indiscriminate use of physical therapy for the relief of symptoms only is not indicated. Transcutaneous stimulation will be satisfactory therapy for about one-third of these patients. Reoperation is indicated only for specific problems that obviously can be corrected. There is little evidence that simply removing scar again is of value to these patients for more than a short period of time. Correction of defective incisions, demonstrated instability, and complete block of cerebrospinal fluid circulation all appear to be worthwhile. Extensive microsurgical procedures for arachnoiditis are indicated, but only when all of the modalities have failed and usually are reserved for patients with progressive or serious neurological deficits.

The use of implantable electrical stimulators for the relief of pain in the chronic low back cripple is also employed. The technique requires percutaneous procedures for testing efficacy. Patients are chosen on the basis of their response to percutaneous spinal cord stimulation. The success of these devices now exceeds 70% in three- to five-year followups, although technical limitations make appropriate patient selection extremely important.

In addition to the specific things that can be done for the chronic low back cripple, it is well to completely evaluate the patient's psychiatric status. Normal patients routinely become depressed and develop chronic anxiety with unremitting, untreated pain. They very often suffer from inactivity and very often become addicted to drugs prescribed by their physicians. These problems need to be treated. In the face of unrelieved drug addiction and severe depression, virtually every therapeutic modality will fail. It is important to treat depression and anxiety appropriately and to eliminate drug addiction. All narcotics should be withdrawn gradually over 7 to 14 days and barbiturates and diazepam should be eliminated. Diazepam accentuates depression and potentially intensifies musculoskeletal pain states. Depression is usually easily treated with a tricyclic. Drugs in common use are doxepin, 75 to 100 mg at bedtime, or amitriptyline, 75 to 100 mg at bedtime. Larger doses may be used. The tricyclics will treat depression over a several week period and will provide normal sleep rapidly in two to four days. Withdrawal effects are commonly treated by diphenhydramine, 25 mg 3 times a day for autonomic symptoms and hydroxyzine pamoate for the agitation and anxiety which so often accompany narcotic withdrawal. Clonidine, 0.1 mg bid to 0.2 mg qid, can be used to reduce the autonomic symptoms associated with withdrawal. As soon as these problems are solved, it is possible to assess pain therapies and the general measures described can then be utilized effectively.

The psychological evaluation should go further than this. The effects of drug addiction and depression are important in normal patients. However, a large number of patients suffering from chronic pain did not begin with a normal premorbid state. A marked percentage suffer from real psychiatric disease such as conversion reaction, post traumatic neurosis, or endogenous depression. An even larger percentage magnify their pain response based upon their personality type. Such patients may exhibit an organic brain syndrome, a preexisting personality disorder, or may magnify their pain as a result of situational stress. This situational stress is usually job related, but it also may be related to family problems or litigation. It is extremely important to obtain an adequate sociological and psychological evaluation of the patient early in the treatment of the chronic low back syndrome. Certainly, no procedures should be undertaken until these data are available. Appropriate therapy for patients with real psychiatric disease is obviously not surgical but psychotherapeutic. Patients who magnify their pain state and unconsciously exaggerate the disability from relatively minor somatic problems usually require behavioral therapy. Unfortunately, in our experience, there is little difference in terms of the number of operations or drugs used in patients with real psychiatric disease, those with behavioral abnormalities, and those with real organic pain states. The identification of these psychological and psychiatric factors early in the course of any chronic pain state is extremely important so that appropriate therapy may be applied and potentially dangerous and ineffectual therapies denied. The patients with psychological and psychiatric problems very often will insist upon surgical therapies and drug therapies. Patient insistence is not an indication for a procedure and the physician must be firm in directing the patient to appropriate therapy.

Related Specific Syndromes That Require Therapy

There are several syndromes that are relatively easy to recognize that present with back pain. It is unusual for the patients not to have neurological deficits and the diagnosis generally presents no difficulty. The first of these is spinal stenosis. The classic symptom of spinal stenosis is pseudoclaudication. These patients have pain and weakness in the legs after exertion. However, the problem is compression of the cauda equina, not vascular insufficiency. The diagnosis is made by myelography, but the suspicion is raised in a patient with the claudication syndrome who has normal pulses in the lower extremities.

The second problem which is considerably more serious than straightforward disc herniation is that of lumbar spondylolysis. The spinal stenosis syndrome may be a part of this larger syndrome or it may be a congenitally acquired state. In lumbar spondylolysis there is degeneration of multiple discs with changes in bone and ligament. The patient usually presents with back pain but with neurological deficits related to multiple root involvement. If untreated, the syndrome may lead to profound neurological deficit, even paraplegia. The plain x-ray films give a clue to the diagnosis since generalized degenerative and hypertrophic changes will be found. Treatment for both spinal stenosis and other degrees of lumbar spondylolysis is decompressive laminectomy, removal of discs which are significantly compressing neural elements, and fusion if significant instability exists. Intraspinal tumors and arteriovenous malformation may also be confused with these pain states and are important in the differential diagnosis. The spinal arteriovenous malformation often presents with low back pain or an intermittent claudication syndrome. Back pain may be an early sign of intraspinal tumor. It is particularly common with intramedullary tumors in the thoracic region and may precede neurological deficits by a long period of time. Until the signs and symptoms become profound, there is little to distinguish the spinal cord tumor from the other spinal syndromes that have been described, and all patients with the chronic back pain problem who have myelography should have the lower conus area investigated thoroughly.

Another matter of interest is the occurrence of arachnoid cysts in the lumbar region in the presence of a complaint of spine pain. It is generally believed that these root cysts do not cause pain and are normally present in many asymptomatic people. However, occasionally one may be large enough to be compressive. In our experience, the ones that are compressive often do not fill on myelography and a clue to the diagnosis is seen because of bony erosion visible on plain x-ray films. A preoperative diagnosis of tumor is often made, and the arachnoid cyst is discovered at the time of surgery.

Summary

The complaint of back pain is one of the most common reasons why patients see physicians in the United States today. Most of the problems do not relate to degenerative disc disease, but are clearly related to obesity, inactivity, and lack of muscle tone. Any program of back care must include correction of these factors. The back pain complaint is currently fashionable in disability and litigation circles as well. It is a legitimate reason to cease work and to recover damages. For this reason, low back pain has been chosen by a large number of patients to serve as an expression of psychiatric disease or situational stress. It is quite probable that such patients do have discomfort, but the underlying problem which makes the disability great and magnifies the discomfort is psychological and not physiological. These factors must be carefully evaluated in planning a therapy program. Specifically, interventional procedures are not warranted. Much of the chronic low back cripple syndrome as it exists today in the United States is because of operations on the lumbar spine, inappropriately applied to patients in these latter categories. Operative procedures should be limited to those individuals with clear-cut herniated intervertebral discs, straightforward syndromes such as spinal stenosis, lumbar spondylolysis or situations in which clear-cut instability exists. Operative procedures for nebulous diagnoses and degenerative disc disease without these specific indications are not indicated and cause notable disability and cost in the United States.

5 Psychological Testing for Chronic Pain Patients

Mary Cowan Viernstein

There is persuasive evidence in the literature of chronic pain that psychological variables correlate with subjective estimates of pain and with treatment outcomes. Bond and Pearson[1] found that in a group of patients with advanced cancer of the cervix those without pain received higher scores on a measure of extraversion and lower scores on a neuroticism measure than the patients with pain. Other investigators report that experience of pain is correlated with degree of neuroticism or other personality variables.[2-7] Hendler et al[8] report personality differences in responders versus nonresponders in electromyographic (EMG) biofeedback treatment. Forrest et al[9] compared good versus poor responders for low back pain treatment and found that depression was an underlying variable for the poor response group. Blumetti and Modesti[10] state the need for a vigorous search for relevant psychological variables due to the high incidence of treatment failure in low back pain. In investigating a group of recipients of treatment for low back pain, they found that improved patients received scores significantly lower on the Hypochondriasis and Hysteria scales of the Minnesota Multiphasic Personality Inventory (MMPI) and on a dependency measure of the Rorschach inkblot test than did the unimproved patients. Erickson et al[11] found that psychological criteria were extremely helpful in selection of patients for implantable stimulators. A study of social modeling influences on psychophysical judgments of electrical stimulation carried out by Craig et al,[12] (1972) presented data relating pain tolerance to age, sex, and race.

Psychological profiles of pain patients have also been found to differ from those of persons without chronic pain.[13-18]

Major difficulties with many psychological studies of chronic pain patients have been the lack of adequate classification of pain patients into appropriate subgroups, the small number of subjects in the studies (from 30 to 50 subjects are needed for analysis of personality data, and results for women and men must be analyzed separately), the lack of an adequate battery of psychological tests, and the lack of cross-validation groups. These difficulties must be addressed to gain further insight into the phenomenon of chronic pain, and thus to refine current pain taxonomies. Ultimately, it is hoped, this will enable us to improve strategies of diagnosis and treatment.

Personality Assessment

It is important to realize that all psychological tests are samples of behavior. They are measurement devices designed to assess some aspect of an individual's personality, and since they are instruments to assess personality, all have an implicitly defined theory of personality. For example, the MMPI[19] assumes the validity of classifying patients according to a system of diagnosis related to Kraepelin's psychiatric classification. Thus, in choosing which psychological tests to assess patients with chronic pain, it is important to formulate clearly which aspects of the patients' personalities you wish to investigate, and then to choose appropriate tests.

The types of tests chosen will also depend upon practical concerns; eg, self-report inventories are more desirable than projective tests from the point of view of time involved in administering and scoring. However, it is important to be certain that a self-report inventory has been keyed adequately with respect to other criteria, so that the scores are not based on how the patient sees himself or herself, but rather reflect externally validated criteria. This has not always been the case.

Historically, methods of personality assessment have included astrology, palmistry, and phrenology, and at present include direct observation of behavior, gathering of biographical data, self-report inventories, and projective techniques.[20] Classification of personality assessment instruments is made in terms of the method of test construction, eg, rational and/or empirical, the aim of the test, and the method of administering the test (self-report, or observer-administered). The purposes of personality testing include increased understanding of psychological data, measurement of individual and group differences, and practical application of test results, eg, selection of individuals for a given purpose.[21]

Current controversy in the field of personality assessment concerns the relative contribution of situational and personality variables to social behavior as well as the actual meaning of variables that are measured by personality testing.[22-28] In a masterful review, Hogan et al[28] presented evidence for the empirical utility of personality testing. They further argued that personality testing should not be viewed from a platonic perspective as an attempt to measure enduring entities inside people (often called "traits"), but rather from an empirical perspective in which the process of measurement consists of applying numbers to responses to test items according to predetermined rules, thereby forming scale scores that are reliable and valid. Thus, in a useful test individuals tend to receive the same scores at different times, there exists a distribution in scores within a given group, and variations in scores are related in meaningful ways with other test scores.

The author believes that it is the latter perspective that is most helpful to persons involved in the psychological testing of patients with chronic pain. Any measure (test) used must be reliable, ie, scores must be consistent and stable, and it must be valid, ie, capable of achieving the aims for which it is employed. "Consistency" and "stability" refer respectively to form-associated and time-associated reliability; both describe the agreement to be expected among similar measurements. There are three types of validity coefficients:

1. Content, referring to how well the test samples the subject matter of the test.
2. Criterion (predictive and concurrent), referring to how well the test estimates the future or current position or rank of the person taking the test with respect to a variable that is external to the test.
3. Construct, referring to how well variables measured by the test relate to variables external to the test in a predictable way (essentially a check on the underlying theory of the test, and usually done to increase one's understanding of what the test is measuring).

Once we have ascertained that a given test is reliable and valid, the appropriateness of using it must be examined thoroughly. For patients with chronic pain, appropriate psychological tests are those which increase our understanding of the patient's psychological state, and improve patient management by aiding in selection of patients for various treatments, eg, surgery, electrical stimulation of the nervous system, psychotherapy, physical therapy, and biofeedback. As Long[29] has emphasized, ". . . the key to successful chronic pain management is to match the patient with the optimal treatment modality." Psychological testing can be a potent tool in the task of matching individual patients with treatments.

This chapter will discuss some of the psychological tests most frequently used in the field of chronic pain, and will present others that have practical advantage for testing patients with chronic pain.

The Minnesota Multiphasic Personality Inventory

The Minnesota Multiphasic Personality Inventory[19] is a self-report inventory consisting of 550 affirmative statements to which the subject responds "true," "false," or "cannot say." It is the most widely used personality inventory in the field of personality assessment and in the psychological evaluation of patients with pain. It provides scores on the following clinical scales:

- Hypochondriasis
- Depression
- Hysteria
- Psychopathic deviate
- Masculinity-femininity
- Paranoia
- Psychasthenia
- Schizophrenia
- Hypomania
- Social introversion

Interpretations of MMPI results must be made using the pattern of the scores on these scales, rather than individual scores. Hendler et al[30] discussed conflicting evidence regarding the utility of the MMPI in predicting treatment outcome, pointing out that the use of the MMPI in selection of treatment for patients with chronic pain appears problematical. Anastasi[21] discussed inherent limitations in the MMPI due to poor reliability and validity. She stated that MMPI scales reflect categories now considered obsolescent and their value in differential diagnosis is questionable. Further, she pointed out that MMPI scales were developed by comparing responses of each clinical group with normal subjects, rather than comparing the responses with those of other clinical groups—the preferred method for differential diagnosis. She noted a further limitation of the MMPI that the standard scores used in deriving profile codes are based on the scores of a small, unrepresentative normative sample (700 Minneapolis adults).

The extensive MMPI data collected and the vast clinical use of the MMPI make it important to test subjects with the MMPI as well as other personality inventories, but one must remember its inherent limitations.

The McGill/Melzack Pain Questionnaire, Part 2

The McGill/Melzack Pain Questionnaire,[31] Part 2 consists of 20 sets of adjectives that describe pain. Subjects circle words in each set that best describe their pain. The questionnaire provides quantitative measures of clinical pain, and appears to have potential for selecting the best alternatives among different methods to relieve pain.[31]

The Symptom Check List-90

The Symptom Check List-90 (SCL-90)[32] is a 90-question, self-report inventory that yields measures of depression, anxiety, somatic concern, self-esteem, hostility, and obsessional thoughts. It measures changes in these personality variables over time, and appears to be useful for testing patients with chronic pain.[30,32]

The Mini-Mental Status Exam

The Mini-Mental Status Exam[33] is a short test of intelligence in which the subject is asked questions such as the current day of the month and his or her present location, and to copy a simple design. It is extremely useful in differentiating organic and psychiatric disease and in identifying persons on the low end of the intelligence-quotient spectrum.

The Adjective Check List

The Adjective Check List (ACL)[34] is a set of 300 adjectives. Subjects are asked to describe themselves in terms of these adjectives by checking those adjectives that describe themselves; this task is usually completed within 10 or 15 minutes. The inoffensiveness of the items makes this an attractive assessment device. The ACL assesses self-concepts and can be scored for such characteristics as self-confidence, self-control, personal adjustment, need for achievement, dominance, affiliation, and autonomy. It is particularly useful for testing of normal populations.

The California Psychological Inventory

The California Psychological Inventory (CPI)[35] is a list of 480 items designed to assess personality characteristics that are important in everyday social interaction. Scores on the CPI reflect how a person will be described by others who know him or her well, and is designed for use primarily with normal subjects. The scales are grouped into four broad categories:

1. Measures of poise and interpersonal adequacy.
2. Measures of socialization and responsibility.
3. Measures of achievement potential and intellectual efficiency.
4. Measures of intellectual and interest modes.

It is one of the better personality inventories available today, and has been useful in such diverse research areas as delinquency, high-level achievement, alcoholism, and vocational guidance.

The Hendler Ten-Minute Screening Test for Chronic Back Pain Patients Hendler's Taxonomy

Hendler[30,36,37] presented a persuasive classification of chronic pain patients into the following four subgroups:

1. The Objective Pain Patient (OPP).
2. The Undetermined Pain Patient (UPP).
3. The Exaggerating Pain Patient (EPP).
4. The Associative Pain Patient (APP).

The two dimensions upon which these classifications are formed are premorbid adjustment and organic etiology of pain. The Objective Pain Patient has good premorbid adjustment, with a known organic basis for the pain. He or she may have psychological problems resulting from the chronic pain. The psychological profile or adjustment of this patient usually depends upon the amount of time he or she has had chronic pain. Within a period of three to twelve years, the OPP has passed through stages of depression and withdrawal, has "learned to live with the pain," and is a productive member of society. The Undetermined Pain Patient also has a good psychiatric and sociological premorbid adjustment, but the organic basis of the UPP's pain is unknown. The UPP passes through the same psychological stages of difficulties and adjustment as the OPP. The Exaggerating Pain Patient has a definite organic basis for his or her chronic pain, but the effect of the pain on the EPP's life is magnified and the EPP's premorbid adjustment is poor. Some subtypes of EPPs are: patients with organic mental disorders or paranoid schizophrenia, drug abusers, patients with psychosomatic pain (eg, patients having muscle tension as the result of anxiety), patients with dependent, compulsive, or histrionic personalities, and patients with Briquet's syndrome (hysterical disorder or hypochondriasis with multiple somatic complaints). EPPs usually resist withdrawal from drugs, complain profusely about their pains, and often experience important secondary gain due to their pain. Associative Pain Patients have poor premorbid adjustment and no apparent organic basis for their pains. Patients with conversion hysteria or psychosis who perceive pain due to disordered thinking are included in this category, as are malingerers.

These categories are useful in predicting whether a patient may benefit from various treatments such as participation in a pain treatment center, psychiatric therapy, or surgical procedures.[30,36,38]

The Hendler Screening Test[30,36] is a 15-item questionnaire designed to classify patients with chronic back and limb pain into the categories described above.* Low scores signify classification as an Objective or Undetermined Pain Patient, midrange scores, classification as Exaggerating Pain Patient, and high scores, classification as an Affective Pain Patient.

Hendler et al[30] and Viernstein et al[17] have reported encouraging reliability and validity for this test. Although further research is necessary, it appears to be a most promising instrument for use in the psychological classification of patients with chronic pain.

Other tests that may be of some use in investigating the personality of the chronic pain patient include projective tests such as the Thematic Apperception Test (TAT), the Pain Apperception Test (Pat), and Rorschach.[20,21] Difficulties in administering and scoring such tests make them less desirable than those discussed here.

As Blumer[39] has so eloquently demonstrated, a thorough psychological evaluation must be made of any patient who presents with the

*For further information concerning this test, address inquiries to Nelson Hendler, MD, Mensana Clinic, Greenspring Valley Road, Stevenson, MD 21153.

complaint of chronic pain before any decisions about treatment are made. Evaluation should be made by means of a psychiatric consultation, an adequate battery of psychological tests, eg, the MMPI, the CPI, and the Hendler Screening Test, and demographic, social, and medical data. Future work in the field of chronic pain must include the development of criteria for determining success or failure of treatment, using such measures as ratings from patients, physicians, psychologists, and nurses, as well as additional follow-up data. The effectiveness of different treatments should be tested in order to improve treatment of pain patients by developing methods of assigning patients to appropriate subgroups.

Ultimately, the characteristics of various subgroups of chronic pain patients must be described in terms of demographic, psychological, cognitive, and medical data. The final criterion for the employment of such subgroups is, of course, improved treatment outcome in the management of patients with chronic pain.

REFERENCES

1. Bond MR, Pearson IB: Psychological aspects of pain in women with advanced cancer of the cervix. *J Psychosom Res* 1969;13:13–19.
2. Merskey H, Boyd D: Emotional adjustment and chronic pain. *Pain* 1978; 5:173–178.
3. Merskey H, Spear FG: *Pain: Psychological and Psychiatric Aspects.* London, Bailliere, Tindall and Cassell, 1967.
4. Sternbach RA: *Pain: A Psychophysiological Analysis.* New York, Academic Press, 1968.
5. Sternbach RA: *Pain Patients: Traits and Treatment.* New York, Academic Press, 1974.
6. Sternbach RA: Psychological factors in pain, in Bonica JJ, Albe-Fessard D (eds): *Advances in Pain Research and Therapy.* New York, Raven Press, 1976, vol 1, pp 293–299.
7. Cox GB, Chapman R, Black RG: The MMPI and chronic pain: The diagnosis of psychogenic pain, to be published.
8. Hendler N, Derogatis L, Avella J, et al: EMG biofeedback in patients with chronic pain. *Dis Nerv Sys* 1977;38:505–509.
9. Forrest AJ, Wolkind SN: Masked depression in men with low back pain. *Rheumatol Rehabil* 1974;13:148–153.
10. Blumetti AE, Modesti LM: Psychological predictors of success or failure of surgical intervention for intractable back pain, in Bonica JJ, Albe-Fessard D (eds): *Advances in Pain Research and Therapy.* New York, Raven Press, 1976, vol 1, pp 323–325.
11. Erickson DL, Michaelson MA, Acharya A: Pain patient selection for implantable stimulating devices, in Bonica JJ, Albe-Fessard D (eds): *Advances in Pain Research and Therapy.* New York, Raven Press, 1976, vol 1, pp 479–482.
12. Craig KD, Best H, Ward LM: Social modeling influences on psychophysical judgments of electrical stimulation. *J Abnorm Soc Psychol* 1975; 84:366–373.

13. Woodrow KM, Friedman GD, Siegelamb AB, et al: Pain tolerance: Differences according to age, sex and race. *Psychosom Med* 1972;34:548–556.
14. Jamison K, Ferrer-Brechner MT, Brechner VL, et al: Correlation of personality profile with pain syndrome, in Bonica JJ, Albe-Fessard D (eds): *Advances in Pain Research and Therapy.* New York, Raven Press, 1976; vol 1, pp 317–321.
15. Sternbach RA, Wolf SR, Murphy RW, et al: Traits of pain patients: The low back "loser." *Psychosomatics* 1973;14:226–229.
16. Harrison RH: Psychological testing in headache: A review. *Headache* 1975;13:177–185.
17. Viernstein MC, Gucer P, Black RG, et al: Personality characteristics of patients with chronic pain. *Pain Abstracts.* Second World Congress on Pain. International Association for the Study of Pain. Seattle, WA, 1978.
18. Henryk-Gutt R, Rees WL: Psychological aspects of migraine. *J Psychosom Res* 1973;17:141–153.
19. Hathaway SR, McKinley JC: *Minnesota Multiphasic Personality Inventory: Manual for Administration and Scoring.* New York, Psychological Corporation, 1967.
20. Lanyon RL, Goodstein LD: *Personality Assessment.* New York, Wiley and Sons, 1971.
21. Anastasi A: *Psychological Testing.* New York, Macmillan and Company, 1976.
22. Mischel W: *Personality and Assessment.* New York, John Wiley, 1968.
23. Mischel W: On the future of personality measurement. *Am Psychol* 1977; 32:246–254.
24. Bandura A: *Social Learning Theory.* Moristown, NJ, General Learning Press, 1971.
25. Harré R, Secord PF: *The Explanation of Social Behavior.* Totowa, NJ, Littlefield, Adams, 1973.
26. Nisbett RE, Caputo C, Legant P, et al: Behavior as seen by the actor and as seen by the observer. *J Person Soc Psychol* 1973;27:154–164.
27. Hogan R, Mankin D, Conway J, et al: Personality correlates of undergraduate marijuana use. *J Consult Clin Psychol* 1970;35:58–63.
28. Hogan R, De Soto CB, Solano C: Traits, tests, and personality research. *Am Psychol* 1977;32:255–264.
29. Long DM: Chronic pain: Staging and stimulation, in Bonica JJ, Melzack R, Liebeskind JC, Nyhus LM, Long CM (eds): *Altering the Experience of Pain.* New York, Pfizer, Inc 1979, pp 29–33.
30. Hendler N, Viernstein MC, Gucer P, et al: New diagnostic categories and a preoperative screening test for chronic back pain patients. *Psychosom Med* 1979;20:800–808.
31. Melzack R: The McGill pain questionnaire: Major properties and scoring methods. *Pain* 1975;1:277–299.
32. Derogatis LR, Rickels K, Rock A: The SCL 90 and the MMPI: A step in the validation of a new self-reporting scale. *Br J Psychiatry* 1976; 128:280–289.
33. Folstein M, Folstein S, McHugh P: Mini-Mental State: A practical method for grading the cognitive state of patients for the clinician. *J Psychiat* 1975;12:189–198.
34. Gough HG, Heilbrun AB: *The Adjective Check List Manual.* Palo Alto, CA, Consulting Psychologists Press, 1965.
35. Gough HG: *Manual for the California Psychological Inventory.* Palo Alto, CA, Consulting Psychologists Press, 1969.
36. Hendler N: Psychiatric considerations of chronic pain, in Youmans JR (ed): *Neurological Surgery.* Philadelphia, WB Saunders Co, 1982.

37. Hendler N: *Diagnosis and Non-Surgical Management of Chronic Pain.* New York, Raven Press, 1981.
38. Long DM, Hendler N, Viernstein MC: Rehabilitation of patients suffering from chronic pain, in Ilis LS, Sedgwick EM, Glanville HJ (eds): *Rehabilitation of the Neurological Patient,* Boston, Blackwell Scientific Publications, 1982, pp 282–311.
39. Blumer D: Psychiatric considerations in pain, in Rothman RH, Simeone FA (eds): *The Spine.* Philadelphia, WB Saunders Co, 1975, pp 871–906.

6 Electrodiagnostic Studies in the Evaluation of Pain

Henry A. Spindler
Marcel A. Reischer

Electrodiagnostic studies are commonly of great value in the evaluation of pain syndromes. The most useful of these studies are electromyography (EMG) and nerve conduction studies (NCS). The purpose of this chapter is to briefly describe these two studies and to detail their use in the evaluation of pain.

The primary function of electromyography and nerve conduction studies is to examine the integrity of the motor unit, which is the basic component of the peripheral nervous system. The motor unit consists of the anterior horn cell, its axon and branches, the neuromuscular junction, and all the muscle fibers which are innervated by that cell. Electromyography and nerve conduction studies can frequently localize a lesion to a particular site in the motor unit and thus diagnose or confirm the presence of a lesion causing a neuromuscular pain syndrome.

ELECTROMYOGRAPHY

Electromyography is the technique of recording voltage changes within a muscle. This electrical activity is displayed on an oscilloscope and monitored through a loudspeaker. The muscle is examined during needle electrode insertion with the muscle completely at rest and during various grades of active muscle contraction.

Response to Needle Electrode Insertion

During electrode insertion there is a short burst of electrical activity followed by silence. In either neuropathic or myopathic disease, increase in the duration of this insertional activity may be the earliest or only sign of abnormality. Decrease in insertional activity indicates a loss of muscle tissue and is usually a late finding in neuromuscular disease.

Muscle at Rest

With the needle electrode resting in relaxed muscle, there is usually electrical silence. Fibrillation potentials are the electrical activity produced by the spontaneous depolarization of a single muscle fiber. These are generally not found in normal muscle and indicate loss of anatomic or physiologic control of the muscle fiber by the motor axon which innervates it. Fibrillation potentials are seen most commonly in neuropathic disease but may also be seen with myopathy.

Positive sharp waves have the same significance as fibrillation potentials. They are felt to originate in single muscle fibers which have been damaged by the needle insertion and which are spontaneously depolarizing.

Fasciculation potentials are the electrical activity generated by an entire motor unit firing spontaneously and not under voluntary control. They are most frequently associated with anterior horn cell disease but may be present in radiculopathy or peripheral neuropathy. Occasionally, fasciculations may be seen in otherwise normal muscle.

Voluntary Muscular Contraction

As muscle contraction begins, motor units are recruited in proportion to the strength of contraction required. The normal motor unit potential contains up to four phases. With five or more phases present, the potential is termed polyphasic. A small proportion of the motor unit potentials present in a normal muscle may be polyphasic, but an increase in this percentage is considered abnormal. Increased numbers of polyphasic motor unit potentials may be seen with either neuropathic or myopathic disease.

The duration of the motor unit potential is from 5 to 12 msec. Increase in this duration is frequently seen in neuropathic disease, while decrease in the duration of the motor unit action potential is commonly associated with myopathic disease. The amplitude of a motor unit action potential generally ranges from 500 μv to 5 mv. Increase in this amplitude is associated with neuropathic disease, while decrease in the amplitude is commonly seen with myopathic disease. These motor unit parameters must be considered generalizations, since they vary with the size of the motor unit being examined and the stage of the neuromuscular disease.

As the strength of voluntary contraction increases in a normal muscle, the number of motor units recruited increases proportionately until individual motor unit potentials can no longer be discerned on the oscilloscope. With maximal voluntary contraction the oscilloscope is completely obscured by the electrical activity, and this is termed a "complete interference pattern." In neuropathic disease where the number of motor units available has decreased, the interference pattern will be incomplete at maximal contraction; in severe cases, individual motor unit potentials will be discernible. In myopathies there is loss of muscle fibers within a motor unit, causing decreased strength within that unit. Therefore, for a fixed strength of contraction, more motor units must be recruited than in normal muscle. This causes a complete interference pattern to occur with a much weaker contraction than in ordinary muscle.

NERVE CONDUCTION STUDIES

Nerve conduction studies involve measuring the time required for an impulse to be carried over a fixed distance of nerve or determining the actual conduction velocity. These studies also involve examining the evoked electrical response in the muscle supplied by the motor nerve or of the actual potential in the sensory fibers.

In motor conduction studies recording electrodes are placed over a muscle supplied by the nerve being studied. The time from stimulation to the onset of the evoked response in the muscle is termed the latency. Nerve conduction velocities are obtained by stimulating the nerve at several points along its length.

Sensory conduction studies are performed by placing recording electrodes directly over the nerve being studied. The nerve is then stimulated proximally, and the time required for the stimulus to reach the recording electrodes is determined.

Slowing of nerve conduction most commonly occurs in diseases of the myelin but may also occur with disease affecting the large, rapidly conducting axons. Nerve conduction may be abnormal with either primary disorders of the nerve or secondary to trauma or local compression.

Any peripheral motor or sensory nerve which is accessible to stimulation and recording may be studied. In the upper extremity motor conduction studies are commonly done on the median, ulnar, and radial nerves, but the axillary and suprascapular nerve may also be studied. Sensory conduction in the upper extremities can be evaluated in the median, ulnar, radial, and medial and lateral antebrachial cutaneous nerves. In the lower extremities motor conduction studies are commonly done in the peroneal, tibial, and femoral nerves. Sensory studies normally are performed on the sural, superficial peroneal, saphenous, medial and lateral plantar nerves, and the lateral femoral cutaneous nerve.

"H" reflex and "F" wave studies are a third form of nerve conduction study used to evaluate the proximal segments of nerve which are inaccessible to standard stimulation techniques. The H reflex is normally only present in the tibial nerve. The tibial nerve is stimulated at the knee with recordings made from the gastrocnemius or soleus. The impulse is carried proximally in the sensory fibers to the spinal cord, where they synapse with the α-motor neurons and are conducted back to the muscle via the α-motor neurons. This reflex study is, therefore, a measure of the integrity of the motor and sensory roots. The F wave is commonly studied in the peroneal, tibial, median, and ulnar nerves. Electrical stimulation is applied to the peripheral nerve with the recording from a distal muscle. The impulse is carried proximally to the spinal cord by the α-motor neurons. There, they cause retrograde firing of the anterior horn cells. These impulses are then carried peripherally again by the α-motor neurons and cause discharge of the muscle fibers which they innervate. Thus, the F-wave study examines only the motor fibers. If an H reflex latency or F-wave latency is prolonged while conduction in the distal motor or sensory nerve fibers is normal, it can be assumed that there is pathology in the proximal segments of the nerve.

For a more detailed discussion of the physiology and techniques of electromyography and nerve conduction studies, the reader is referred to one of the standard texts.[1-3]

CLINICAL APPLICATIONS

Radiculopathies

Cervical and lumbar radiculopathies are very common causes of musculoskeletal pain. These may appear as radiating pain into the extremity with associated paresthesias and weakness. If the root lesion is causing damage to the motor fibers within the root, EMG abnormalities may be seen in muscles supplied by that root. By examining muscles representing each of the nerve roots supplying an extremity, the electromyographer may be able to localize the lesion to a single root or determine that multiple levels are involved. In radiculopathy the earliest EMG abnormalities are frequently and only in the paraspinal musculature. In addition to indicating that an abnormality is present, findings in the paraspinal musculature indicate that the lesion is at least as proximal as the posterior primary ramus and usually indicates a root level lesion.

Electromyography may, however, be normal in the presence of a radiculopathy. Since it requires three to four weeks following nerve injury for fibrillations to appear, an examination performed before this time may be normal. If abnormalities then appear on a repeat examination after this time period has elapsed, the approximate time of onset of the lesion can be documented. This is frequently helpful in a medical-legal context and when the patient has a history of multiple past episodes of pain, injury, or surgery. Electromyography may also be normal if the root compression involves only sensory fibers, since EMG will detect only abnormalities in the motor fibers.

Since the peripheral nerves carry fibers from multiple root levels, NCS will generally be normal in a radiculopathy. Only if there is severe involvement of multiple roots with loss of large numbers of motor fibers, will there be abnormalities in standard peripheral NCS. In the presence of an S-1 radiculopathy, the H reflex latency may be prolonged or the H reflex totally absent, since this study depends on the integrity of the motor and sensory fibers in the S-1 root.

In addition to extemity pain, paresthesias, and weakness, radiculopathies may be the cause of axial pain syndromes. Headaches commonly are are associated with upper cervical radiculopathies. Chest pain is not uncommon with cervical radiculopathy, and it should be considered in patients with atypical chest pain who have negative cardiac evaluations.

Thoracic radiculopathies are much less common than cervical or lumbar radiculopathies but may be the cause of noncardiac chest pain or abdominal pain.[3] In patients with abdominal pain but otherwise normal evaluations, a radiculopathy should be considered. This may be secondary to actual root compression but is also commonly seen in diabetics. Pelvic, groin, and testicular pain may also be seen with radiculopathy in the upper lumbar region, and an EMG should be considered when no other cause is found for the symptoms.

Entrapment Syndromes

Peripheral nerve entrapment syndromes are a common cause of pain, weakness, and paresthesias in the extremities.[4] Carpal tunnel syndrome is by far the most common peripheral nerve entrapment syndrome.

However, multiple areas of nerve entrapment exist. Nerves commonly involved in entrapment syndromes include the median nerve at the wrist and elbow, ulnar nerve at the wrist and elbow, suprascapular nerve, femoral nerve, lateral femoral cutaneous nerve, and tibial nerve at the ankle.

The principal finding with nerve conduction testing in entrapment neuropathies is slowing of conduction across the involved segment of nerve, with normal conduction proximal and/or distal to it. Sensory fibers are usually involved first with motor conduction slowing occurring later. Electromyographic abnormalities in the muscles supplied by the entrapped nerve may also be found.

Median nerve Median nerve entrapment at the wrist (carpal tunnel syndrome) usually presents with paresthesias in the median distribution of the hand. However, many patients fail to localize their paresthesias and feel the whole hand is involved. Commonly, there is pain in the hand and wrist, with radiation up the arm to the shoulder. Shoulder pain may be the only symptom, and a cervical radiculopathy may be felt to be present. Weakness in the hand, dropping of small objects, and nocturnal awakening are other common complaints. Electrodiagnostic studies in this condition may show slowing of median sensory and motor conduction across the wrist, with EMG abnormalities in the thenar muscles. Again, sensory conduction abnormalities usually occur first with motor conduction and EMG abnormalities occurring later. In very early carpal tunnel syndrome, all studies may be normal.

The median nerve may also be entrapped in the forearm at the level of the pronator teres (pronator syndrome). This syndrome is much less common than median entrapment at the wrist. Patients with this condition have complaints similar to carpal tunnel syndrome, but pain in the forearm is more prominent. Nerve conduction studies may show slowing of median conduction in the forearm as well as EMG abnormalities in the median innervated forearm musculature.

Ulnar nerve Ulnar nerve entrapment at the elbow is the second most common entrapment syndrome. These patients commonly complain of paresthesias in the ulnar distribution of the hand, weakness in the hand, and pain in the elbow. These symptoms may at times be confused with a C-8 radiculopathy. Nerve conduction studies in these patients commonly show slowing of ulnar motor and sensory conduction across the elbow, with decrease in the amplitude of the ulnar sensory nerve action potential. Electromyographic abnormalities, if present, will be confined to the ulnar innervated musculature. Frequently, only the hand muscles are abnormal since innervation to the forearm muscles from the ulnar nerve frequently occurs proximal to the area of compression.

The ulnar nerve may also be entrapped at the wrist in Guyon's canal. In this case, nerve conduction studies may show prolongation of the ulnar distal sensory and/or motor latency, while proximal conduction will be normal.

While not strictly an ulnar nerve entrapment syndrome, thoracic outlet syndrome frequently presents as pain and paresthesias in the ulnar distribution of the arm and hand. This compression syndrome commonly affects vascular components in the thoracic outlet more than the brachial plexus. However, when nerve conduction abnormalities are present, there will be slowing of ulnar motor conduction through the thoracic outlet. This can be tested with stimulation of the ulnar nerve in the axilla and in the supraclavicular fossa or at the level of the C-7 spinous process. Slowing of ulnar F-wave conduction through the thoracic outlet can also document this syndrome.

Suprascapular nerve Suprascapular nerve entrapment at the scapular notch will result in pain in the shoulder. If severe, there may be atrophy of the supra- and infraspinatus muscles. This nerve entrapment syndrome can easily be misdiagnosed as a C5-6 radiculopathy. However, nerve conduction studies may show slowing in motor conduction of the suprascapular nerve. The EMG is also useful if abnormalities are confined to the supra- and infraspinatus muscle with no abnormalities in any other C5-6 innervated muscles.

Radial nerve While not truly an entrapment syndrome, the radial nerve is frequently compressed in the spinal groove in "Saturday night palsy." These patients develop sudden onset of weakness and numbness in the radial distribution. Radial motor conduction studies will show absence or slowing of radial motor conduction across the spiral groove. Radial sensory conduction may be present or absent, depending on the severity of the compression. Electromyographic abnormalities will be confined to the radial distribution distal to the site of injury.

Again, while not an intrinsic entrapment syndrome, the sensory branch of the radial nerve may be compressed at the wrist by handcuffs, causing pain and paresthesias in the radial distribution of the hand (cheralgia paresthetica). In this case, radial motor conduction studies will be normal, while radial sensory conduction across the wrist will be abnormal. Electromyography will be normal since the compression is distal to the radial motor branches.

Lateral femoral cutaneous nerve The lateral femoral cutaneous nerve may be entrapped at the level of the anterior superior iliac spine, with resultant pain and paresthesias in the lateral aspect of the thigh (meralgia paresthetica). This syndrome may be misdiagnosed as a lumbar radiculopathy. Sensory conduction studies may be abnormal in this nerve. Since the lateral femoral cutaneous nerve is purely sensory, motor studies and electromyography will be normal.

Femoral nerve The femoral nerve may be entrapped at the level of the inguinal ligament, causing pain paresthesias and weakness in the femoral distribution. This entrapment may be confused with an L3-4 radiculopathy. In this syndrome femoral nerve conduction studies may show slowing across the inguinal ligament. Abnormalities of the EMG, if present, will be confined to the femoral nerve distribution.

Peroneal nerve Again, while not strictly an intrinsic entrapment syndrome, the peroneal nerve is subject easily to external compression at the level of the fibular head. This may cause pain, weakness, and paresthesias in the peroneal distribution and may easily be confused with an L-5 radiculopathy. This syndrome may be confirmed by slowing of peroneal motor conduction across the fibular head, decrease or absence of the superficial peroneal sensory nerve action potential, and EMG abnormalities confined to the peroneal distribution rather than an L-5 distribution.

Tibial nerve The tibial nerve may become entrapped at the ankle (tarsal tunnel syndrome). This syndrome frequently causes pain in the ankle, heel, and foot with paresthesias in the toes. Tibial motor conduction studies will show prolongation of the tibial distal motor latency in either the medial or lateral plantar nerves. Sensory abnormalities may also be found in either of these distal branches of the tibial nerve. Abnormalities of the EMG are only of importance if confined to the tibial distribution on the involved side and not present in other intrinsic foot muscles. In any case, EMG abnormalities in the foot muscles must be interpreted with caution, since these muscles are subject to much local trauma in normal individuals.

Peripheral Polyneuropathies

Polyneuropathies may be the cause of diffuse or localized pain, paresthesias, or weakness. Depending on the type of neuropathy, there may be primarly axonal damage with abnormalities seen on EMG and in the parameters of the evoked responses, or the damage may involve primarily the myelin sheath with slowing of conduction. Commonly, both types of abnormality are present. In peripheral polyneuropathies, the lower extremity nerves tend to be affected sooner than the upper, and sensory nerves sooner than motor. The findings tend to be fairly symmetric, but some nerves may be more severely involved than others. In the mononeuritis multiplex type of peripheral neuropathy seen with vasculitis, one nerve may be severely abnormal while others are not markedly affected.

Peripheral neuropathy in diabetics may present in several forms. The most common type shows distal sensory and motor involvement with distal paresthesias and weakness. There is also a form of small fiber diabetic neuropathy which shows no slowing on conduction studies, since in standard studies only conduction in the large fibers can be determined. Diabetic neuropathy also may be present as an acute radicular or plexis neuropathy as seen in "diabetic amyotrophy."

ORDERING THE ELECTRODIAGNOSTIC EXAMINATION

Unlike electrocardiography or electroencephalography, EMG and NCS cannot be performed as routine laboratory procedures. They are an extension of the clinical examination and thus require that a detailed history and physical examination be performed by a physician prior to planning the electrodiagnostic study. The results of the electrical studies must then be interpreted in the light of the clinical findings. This study is a dynamic procedure and cannot be rigidly carried out. A patient may be seen for a possible carpal tunnel syndrome, with the initial emphasis placed on median nerve conduction studies. However, further examination may reveal evidence of other entrapment syndromes, radiculopathies, or peripheral neuropathies requiring alteration of the examination while it takes place. Ideally, the electrodiagnostic study should be performed by a clinical neurophysiologist whose training has met the criteria developed by the American Association of Electromyography and Electrodiagnosis.[5] Unfortunately, in some states, this study may be performed by unsupervised technicians with little medical background.

When requesting an electrodiagnostic study, the training of the examiner must be kept in mind. If the examination is to be performed by a physician-clinical neurophysiologist, it is perhaps best simply to request evaluation of the involved area, ie, upper or lower extremity pain syndrome. If the examination is to be performed by a technician, all of the diagnostic possibilities must be outlined, and the specific nerves and muscles to be tested must be listed. It is not uncommon to see a patient with a diagnosis of possible carpal tunnel syndrome receive only median conduction studies. In this case, a negative or even a positive examination gives very limited information. This would be analogous to referring a patient for a chest roentgenogram to rule out rib fracture, with no attention being given to the soft tissue structures seen on the same x-ray film. With so much valuable information to be gained, the full capabilities of this study should be utilized.

REFERENCES

1. Goodgold J, Eberstein A: *Electrodiagnosis of Neuromuscular Disease,* ed 2. Baltimore, Williams & Wilkins Co, 1977.
2. Lenman LG, Ritchie FM: *Clinical Electromyography.* Philadelphia, Lippincott, 1976.

3. Johnson E: *Practical Electromyography.* Baltimore, Williams & Wilkins Co, 1980.
4. Kopell HP, Thompson WA: *Peripheral Entrapment Neuropathies.* Baltimore, Williams & Wilkins Co, 1963.
5. *Guidelines in EMG.* Rochester, MN, American Association of Electromyography and Electrodiagnosis, 1979.

7 The Use of Thermography in the Diagnosis of Pain Syndromes

Nelson H. Hendler
Cynthia A. Cimini

The use of thermography has gained widespread acceptance in the field of medicine, but for many physicians the entire process is somewhat enigmatic. With the currently available techniques, one can now evaluate the presence or absence of both chronic and acute nerve root irritation, headache, and a variety of vascular disorders. As a diagnostic tool, thermography may well represent an enormous step in the ability to evaluate chronic pain problems.

The word thermogram means a "heat picture." A thermogram is a picture of the heat emitted from the body (see Figures 7-1 and 7-2). No radiation is involved in the process; therefore, there is no hazard to the patient or to the clinician. The thermogram may be a photograph in either black and white or color, or may be obtained using a variety of photographic and recording techniques involving videotape and heat-sensitive paper. The recording techniques can be manipulated so that high-contrast photographs are obtained, demonstrating clear-cut temperature differences, or can be modified so that gradations of temperature may be documented through the use of the tone film.

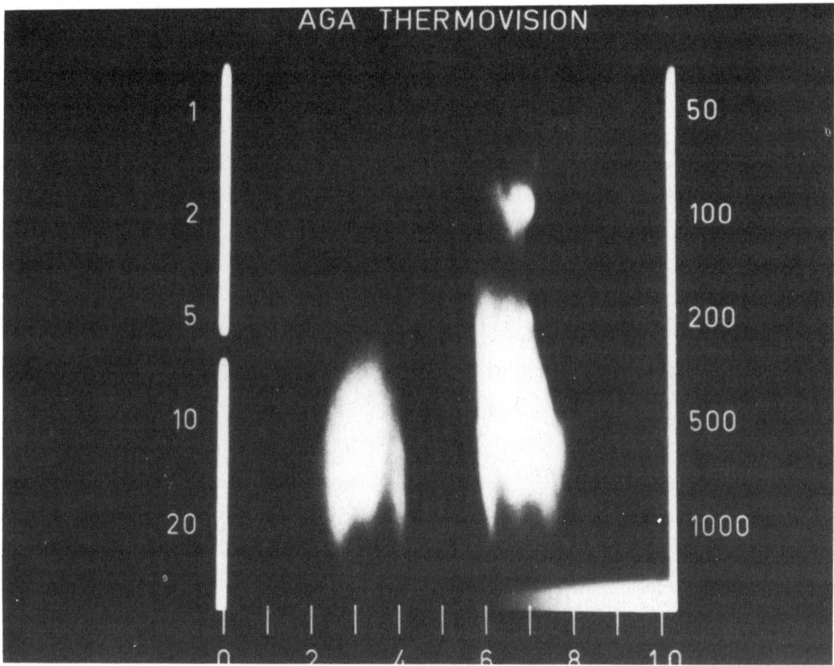

Figure 7-1 This is a thermogram of the hands held upright, indicating that the right hand is 1.5 C colder than the left hand.

Technique

There are two major differences in the techniques for recording temperature changes on the body. The first technique involves a noncontact process, using commercially available thermograph machinery, and the second technique involves the contact of temperature-sensitive material to the skin.

The most critical element in obtaining accurate thermographic recordings of the human body involves the appropriate technique. Without proper technique, improper interpretations and faulty clinical understanding only confound, rather than assist, the physician. Artifacts are legion in thermographic application, so one must be constantly aware of sources of error that can occur. These are most often caused by faulty technique.

There are some basic guides to follow for producing quality thermograms. The climate of the room is critical. The room should be draft free, with maintenance of constant temperature. Drafts can cause artifacts on the thermogram. One of the best mechanisms for climate control is the plenum system. Cold air is forced through an area above the

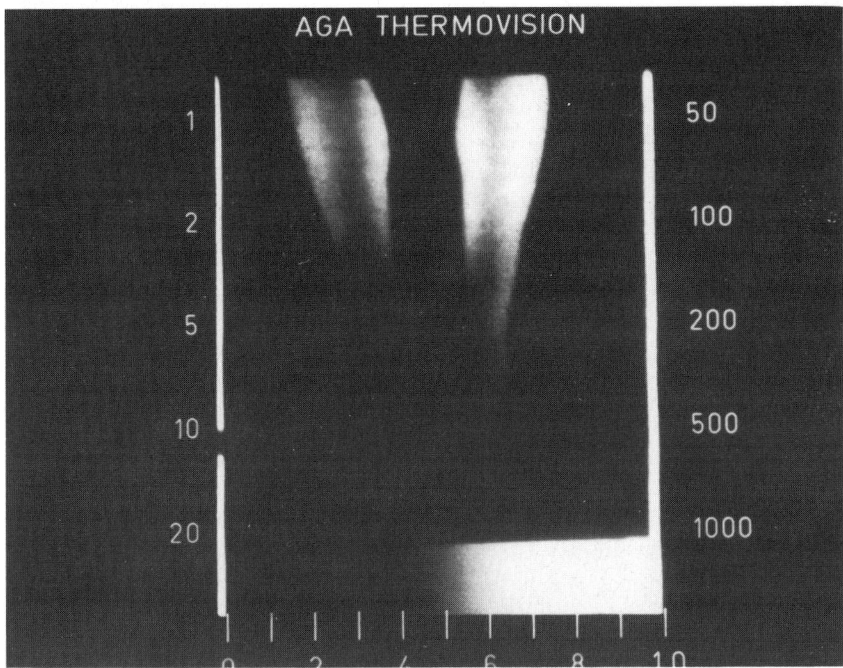

Figure 7-2 This is a thermogram of the legs, indicating that the right leg is 1 C colder than the left leg.

ceiling. This filters down through a porous ceiling, thus producing an even cooling of the room. The draft-free air conditioning system should maintain a constant temperature of 68 to 70 F.

The second critical consideration is the posture of the patient. The skin temperature of the patient should be allowed to equilibrate with the temperature of the room; this normally requires a 10-minute equilibration period. The patient should sit or stand, with the part to be examined totally bare. No part of the body should touch another part of the body, especially in the area to be examined. All jewelry and other apparel should be removed, if possible. Obviously, a leg or arm cast cannot be removed, but elastic bandages, watches, bracelets, rings, eyeglasses, and other artificial adornments are typical causes for artifact production. After the cooling period, the thermographic instrument is either focused or applied to the skin. A corrective middle temperature is of utmost importance, because any change in the setting between examinations eliminates any basis of comparison.

The other important requirement is the establishment of a protocol and technique for measuring and photographing the results obtained with thermographic procedures. This means establishment of a uniform distance between the patient and the thermographic instrument, and/or allowing the liquid crystal material to remain on the skin for a uniform amount of time, at a given and uniform pressure, and with the proper selection of the temperature range.

As mentioned previously, there are two major differences in technique, the noncontact thermographic-infrared equipment, and the contact liquid crystal technique. The liquid crystal technique is more difficult technically. The liquid crystal sheet, containing a heat-sensitive chemical that changes color in response to temperature changes, consists of a rubber sheet impregnated with the crystal. The rubber sheet is then suspended or mounted on a transparent Plexiglas box. The box is filled with air, which produces a positive pressure, and then the sheet is pressed against the body. The sheet is soft and flexible, and thus conforms to the contours of the body. However, this does not always provide adequate contact, especially in areas around the shoulder, head, face, buttocks, and other areas of the body with pronounced curves and indentations. With contact, a color image appears, which represents the heat pattern in that particular area. The image is then photographed, and the photograph produces the permanent record. The type of film used is critical for accurately recording the thermogram, and this will be discussed later.

The liquid crystals utilized for contact thermography are cholesterol derivatives, which selectively reflect polarized light in a narrow region or wave length. They have a strong molecular rotatory power in a specific temperature range which produces the color that is utilized for color thermography. In the past, adaptation of liquid crystals to thermography has been hampered by the need to prepare the skin with a black water-based paint, which was available in a variety of forms. After the black paint had been applied, the liquid crystals were applied to the skin and photographed. Rigid plastic plates replaced skin preparations and spraying, but the lack of flexibility of the plates precluded uniform skin contact, especially when applied to the spine or extremities. As a result, thermographic examination utilizing this technique was woefully inadequate. The use of the flexible rubberized sheet impregnated with crystals has improved the contact thermogram to some degree, but it, too, is fraught with inadequacies, as mentioned above.

The most commonly employed and clinically acceptable technique utilizes an infrared heat measurement technique, utilizing liquid helium as a temperature standard. By utilizing this noncontact method, the instrument to skin artifact is eliminated. This is a serious consideration, since very often the application of a measuring instrument to the surface of the skin may itself alter the skin temperature or electrical resistance, with subsequent change in temperature of the skin. Thermographic equipment is manufactured by a number of companies. One company

(AGA Corp, Secaucus, NJ) manufactures a thermograph in which infrared radiations from the skin are transmitted to the instrument, which then displays the thermographic changes on a television screen. Utilizing various settings on the machine, a single temperature can be requested, and a color will appear indicating what areas of the skin have that particular preset temperature. This technique is called isotherm technique. On the other hand, the instrument can be set in such a way that cold areas of the skin will show as black, and warm areas will show as white. Various gradations can be achieved, especially with the use of appropriate photographic film, which is discussed below. If one area of the body is the painful area, then it is best to compare the temperature in the painful area to a corresponding area of the body on the opposite side. Also, it is most useful to compare the painful area (subjectively reported by the patient) to surrounding body tissue. In this fashion, the thermograph records the temperature changes, as manifested in the skin, associated with the painful process.

The polarity of the final picture, that is, whether hot is represented by white or hot is represented by black, is the subject of much controversy. Early thermographic pictures were associated with x-rays films and for this reason the standard of using black for background and white for information, analogous roentgenograms, was employed as a general technique. However, the use of a white background with black representing hot spots allows the clinician to better visualize the important parts of the image. This concept was borne out by Berreus in experiments conducted in the eighteenth century which showed that the human eye can more easily detect small changes in the black end of the density scale than in the white end. Therefore, if information is displayed in shades of gray and black on a white background, it should be easier to detect and evaluate slight gradations of temperature.

When one photographs the thermographic image, the technique of the recording process is of great importance. Of course, Polaroid film requires no processing. Seventy-mm film produces better images which may be enhanced by altering the process involved in developing the film. However, high-contrast film, which is most useful for radiologists, may not be appropriate for thermography. It is most appropriate to select adequately developed films with a long gray scale. Of course, the uniformity of the development technique is of paramount importance.

Artifacts on the film can produce problems for the clinician. One must be aware of the fact that patients may have disturbed the cooling process by touching parts of their body, scratching themselves, or even leaning against equipment in the room. In order to avoid overinterpreting these artifacts, a patient should always be questioned about the possibility of these movements and noncompliance with instructions if any artifacts appear on the film. This is especially true in patients who may receive workmen's compensation insurance; these patients may attempt to produce painful areas, especially if coached by a well-informed attorney.

In order to achieve optimal and consistent photographic results, the temperature range, central temperature level, resolution, and photographic exposure should be standardized. To facilitate standardization, a test program should be instituted in which the thermographic unit and photographic equipment are checked monthly for temperature range, central temperature calibration, and resolution. Also, a test target, consisting of a Barnes Engineering Thermal Gray Scale, should be photographed for consistency of resolution, utilizing a uniform protocol. After this monthly check, the unit should be adjusted to bring it in line with the specifications, and the test film should be compared with those obtained in preceding months.

The recording techniques for making a permanent thermogram vary quite a bit. One of the techniques utilizes a thermographic scanner, which all seem to be similar in operation, despite the variety available. Mechanical scanners work by either transmission or reflective optics, and recording devices can display or store the thermographic image. One common technique is facsimile transmission, which is used by newspapers and wire services. The image is formed on a rotating drum, after receiving electrical impulses. Chemically treated paper is moved between the drum and the ground bar, creating a "moving spot" effect. By varying the electrical voltage on the drum controls, the amount of current passing through the paper is determined by the temperature of the photographed object. The drum is synchronized with a horizontal scanning system, and the voltage on the drum is modulated by the infrared detector output. Utilizing this facsimile printing, varying shades of gray representing the temperature differences of a patient are produced. There are several advantages to this technique, since it produces a high-quality image with a vast variety of gray tones. Also, the cost of materials is low. Unfortunately, the disadvantages seem to outweigh the advantages, since the process is relatively slow and the images fade after long periods of storage.

Dry silver paper, which is photosensitive and utilizes heat rather than chemicals to develop the image, produces a permanent record. However, this technique is fraught with many technical difficulties, and is not popular.

Most systems now utilize some sort of video or television display, and the resulting image on the cathode ray tube is photographed. This provides a permanent record of the thermogram. Many laboratories utilize Polaroid #107 black-and-white film. This obviously is convenient, requires no developing chemicals or machinery, and the results are immediately available. The drawbacks are the high cost of photographing a large number of patients and/or a large number of photographs per patient. Also, because of the contrast of the film, subtle temperature changes are not perceived, and are difficult to record. Other types of Polaroid film which have excellent gray tones are available, but their cost is even higher.

Some laboratories utilize 70-mm film because of the quality of the picture and the economy. Usually, laboratories that work in conjunction with x-ray film processing laboratories utilize this technique. As a result of the experience in the laboratory of Merlinger,[1] the recommended film is a clear base film, which gives the best gray tones; this is used in preference to a blue-based film. Of the many film types available, Kodak Linograph Shellburst film #2476 (SO-13) seems to have the long gray scale which allows precise resolution of infrared images. Additionally, it is readily machine processed and can be utilized in a bulk loading camera, which has a magazine capable of holding 150 feet of film.

The advent of color thermography has produced a new wave of interest in the process. In color thermography, various shades of gray are electronically translated into different hues or color bands. This makes assessment of different temperatures easy, because the human eye can easily distinguish between different colors. Unfortunately, there are several disadvantages. The capacity for translating small temperature changes into color poses a problem, for example, in breast thermography, because the pattern of vessels is lost in the fields of many colors. In the assessment of allergy, peripheral vascular disease, skin diseases, burns, back pain, limb pain, and other clinical entities in which the quantification of the thermogram is useful, color is a very valuable technique. However, until there are additional refinements, it is best to utilize color thermography in conjunction with black-and-white results.

Video recording of the thermogram is the most common method of producing permanent records. In addition to providing readily accessible material, computer processing of the video image greatly enhances the interpretation. Several manufacturers use video frame storage units so that an image can be frozen and presented on a conventional television monitor for study. One advantage of this technique is that it allows the operator to manipulate the picture quality during the viewing. By changing the image electronically, the best possible characteristics for interpretation can be enhanced.

Clinical Applications

The clinical applications for thermography are myriad, but there are many conflicting reports in the literature. The major cause for concern centers on the overly enthusiastic acceptance of the technique and the overinterpretation of results. Pochaczevsky[2] discussed the use of liquid crystal thermography in the evaluation of spinal root syndromes. He presented data on 114 patients, 63 of whom were hospitalized and had myelograms, and 30 of whom had been operated upon. In comparing the use of conventional infrared thermography with liquid crystal thermography, he found that liquid crystal thermography correlated well with conventional infrared thermography. He felt that liquid crystal thermography had certain advantages, since the entire apparatus is far less expensive than infrared thermography and can be used in doctors' offices and small hospitals. He was especially impressed with the mobility of the apparatus, and the fact that it could be used at the bedside. Unfortunately, he failed to address the various problems attendant upon skin contact processes, and the alteration of skin temperature as a result of the technique.

However, Pochaczevsky[2] did indicate that liquid crystal thermography compared favorably with electromyographic (EMG) or myelographic results. He advocates the use of thermography to screen patients prior to myelography, which may improve selection techniques for this procedure. Also, he advocates the use of thermography as an alternative to EMG or myelographic testing, especially when the latter two are negative.

Pochaczevsky believes that there are a variety of conditions for which liquid crystal thermography is useful. In the evaluation of spondylitis of the spine, and sacroiliac joint assessment, he believes that thermographic changes correspond with complaints of pain. He further advocates its use in diagnosis of deep venous thrombosis, ischemia, rheumatoid arthritis, a temperature-linked sensory loss of leprosy, and stroke. He believes further that the liquid crystal thermography may confirm suspected spinal root compression syndrome associated with herniated disc and osteophyte formation. He has found the technique useful for the detection of spinal canal stenosis, including lateral recess stenosis and subluxation, and hypertrophy of the superior vertebral facets. Additionally, he believes that this technique can graphically demonstrate pain in spinal muscles or in musculoligamentous injuries, while radiographic studies may be normal. The technique may also document the presence of inflammatory processes, infection, and traumatic and peripheral arthropathies. Finally, he suggests that the use of liquid crystal thermography may facilitate monitoring of treatment by providing a baseline measurement, and later a comparison film, after treatment has been effected.

Hendler et al[3] have utilized the standard infrared thermographic technique, to differentiate psychogenic pain from pain with definite organic features. The authors evaluated 224 patients who were referred by orthopedic surgeons, neurosurgeons, or neurologists with a diagnosis of psychogenic pain. The patients were referred to a psychiatrist for evaluation of psychodynamic issues contributing to their pain. It is important to emphasize that the psychiatric diagnosis came from the referring physicians, not from the psychiatrists evaluating them. The 224 patients represented all chronic pain patients referred for psychiatric evaluation to the Chronic Pain Treatment Center at Johns Hopkins Hospital during a 14-month period. A thermogram was considered positive if 1 C temperature difference existed between the area considered painful and the corresponding area on the opposite side or surrounding areas. It was found that 43 of the 224 patients (19%) had abnormal thermograms in the limb in which they complained of pain. The abnormal thermograms were attributable to either reflex sympathetic dystrophy, nerve root irritation, or facet syndrome. This study illustrates the frequency with which an unjustified psychiatric diagnosis is placed upon patients with the subjective complaint of pain, which cannot be documented by EMG, nerve conduction velocity studies, x-ray study, or myelography. Most distressing is the fact that many of the patients had clinical signs and symptoms compatible with their diagnosis, which had either been minimized or neglected by the referring physician, since there was no objective verification of their subjective complaint of pain until thermography was obtained. Therefore, the authors concluded that the use of thermography is useful for validating the complaint of pain in the absence of positive EMG, nerve conduction velocity studies, myelography, cursory physical examinations, and inadequate history taking.

Uematsu and his co-workers,[4] in more extensive study of 803 patients with chronic pain syndrome, found that 54% of these patients (431) had abnormal skin temperature which was documented by thermographic changes of 1 C or greater in measurements. In patients with documented reflex sympathetic dystrophy, when thermography was compared to EMG and nerve conduction velocity findings, only 5 out of 32 cases (16%) had abnormalities on EMG and nerve conduction velocity studies, even though thermography was abnormal. Conversely, when there was clinical, EMG, and nerve conduction velocity verification of a nerve injury, thermography was abnormal in 89% of the cases. The authors believe that thermography appears to be a most effective method of detection for cases with organic pain syndromes and reflex sympathetic dystrophy. This is an important consideration, since early detection of reflex sympathetic dystrophy facilitates its treatment, and prolongation of the diagnosis reduces the change of successful treatment.

Friedman and Wood[5] have written a definitive article on the use of thermography in the diagnosis of headache. The various clinical considerations are covered in Chapter 13, but they will be briefly restated here. The theoretical mechanism behind the pain produced by migraine headache is based on direct observation of the vessels and the response to vasoconstricting agents used during an attack. These observations, associated with other experimental methods including pulse wave recordings and blood flow studies, confirm the vascular basis of these types of headaches. However, one should bear in mind that only 6% of all headache pain is due to migraine per se.

Thermography provides a two-dimensional photographic map of the areas of the face and forehead supplied by the internal and external carotid arteries. Utilizing this technique, isolated areas of heat or cold can be measured, which indicate the relative amount of blood flow into tissues of the skin. Normal facial thermography displays a symmetrical pattern, exhibiting some differences in blood flow around the eyes and mouth. Areas of normal warmth include portions of the face where heat can be trapped, such as the inner canthi and deep skin folds. These appear white on average thermography. The flat portions of the face, particularly the forehead, are relatively even in temperature, and usually present as gray. Cooler areas are the cheeks, nose, and ears, and areas in the head that are insulated by hair: these areas appear black on normal thermography.

Changes in blood flow in the internal or external carotid arteries produce zones of relative warmth or coolness, with a resultant asymmetry. The median supraorbital area is supplied by the ophthalmic arteries, and reflect circulation provided by the internal carotid artery. However, the thermal pattern of the lateral and upper portions of the forehead and most of the face depends on the external carotid arteries.

In a six-year study encompassing 518 patients who underwent thermographic examination, Friedman and Wood[5] found that 78% of these patients were classified as having common and classic migraine headaches, nonmigrainous vascular headaches, muscle contraction headaches, and combined vascular-muscular contraction headaches. One hundred and twelve of these patients were classified as having cluster headache. This does not represent the general headache population, but obviously represents patients seen by the authors.

In cluster headache, there is a unique thermographic pattern, with two-thirds of these patients having coolness in one of the suborbital regions, always on the same side of the headache. These islands of hypothermia appear in the median supraorbital area, which is supplied by the external branches of the internal carotid artery. This abnormality was present in two-thirds of the patients with cluster headache. In many instances, cold spots were also present in the periorbital areas, which are supplied by the external carotid artery. The prominent features of the hypothermic areas in cluster headache were the clear lines of demarcation between the hypothermic area and normal surrounding tissue, and the 1.0 to 1.5 C coolness when compared to these areas. In some cases, coldness was as much as 3 C. The average size of the cold island measured 0.5 cm in diameter on the forehead, but usually was smaller. The pathophysiological basis for cluster headache attacks is not well-known, and the reader is referred to Chapter 13. The proposed mechanism, according to a variety of sources, suggests that there is localized narrowing of the extradural portion of the internal carotid artery during an attack. This narrowing spreads proximally to the upper portion of the carotid canal. Another possible explanation suggests that arteriovenous shunting may occur, and this may cause the pain of cluster headache. Unfortunately, thermography does not differentiate between these two mechanisms. The thermography of cluster headache differs notably from that of migraine headache, in that the former has smaller areas of coldness.

In migraine headache, the entire affected side was colder by approximately 1 C in 75% of the patients studied. However, in 10% of the patients studied, the affected area was warmer, while the forehead recording remained symmetrical in 15% of the cases. When the headache was relieved by ergotamine tartrate, the temperature pattern of the forehead became symmetrical. Interestingly, in patients with cluster headache, the administration of 100 mg of niacin to patients during a cluster headache did not precipitate a headache, nor cause thermographic changes in the supraorbital area, even up to one hour after administration of the drug. Interestingly, papaverine in dosages of 50 mg administered to normal subjects produced an increase in supraorbital skin temperature of approximately 1 C in all individuals examined. Alcohol produced a similar warming of 1 to 2 C.

Among the vasoconstricting agents, Cafregot produced no thermographic changes in either the patients with headache or controls. Likewise, Gynergen produced no change, while Midrin produced minimal cooling in two individuals, but the cold spots of cluster headache were not affected. These findings were the same whether or not the patient was experiencing a headache or free of pain at the time.

One of the more perplexing aspects of evaluating cluster headaches, using thermographic techniques, was the lack of correlation between the objective findings of the thermogram when compared to the clinical activity of the recurring headache. It seems that the cool spots persisted long after the clinically perceived attacks occurred which suggest that changes in the blood vessels, whether they be arteries, arterioles, or even possibly capillaries, are a reflection of a fixed vascular state, and may suggest structural rather than transient vasoconstriction. Based on this evidence, Friedman and Wood[5] propose that the fixed thermographic pattern of cluster headache suggests that factors other than vascular alteration are involved in the production of pain.

Wexler[6] suggests that marked musculoligamentous spasm will also produce relative cold spots in the area of abnormality. However, it has been the author's experience that certain spasms produce actual warm spots in the area of perceived pain. Wexler also indicated that marked and protracted muscle spasm or strain will produce irritation of nerve roots, which may alter interpretation of the results. Importantly, thermography cannot differentiate between herniated disc, muscle spasm, or chronic irritation of the nerve root. Also, there is no way to differentiate the age of the nerve root irritation that might be detected by thermography. This is an important consideration in many medical-legal cases. The only way to lend any temporal validity to thermography obviously occurs if thermograms are done at different points in time, and the change is demonstrable.

Interpretative Precautions

It is important to recognize that thermography does not demonstrate any abnormal anatomic features such as x-ray films might do, but actually demonstrates a physiological change in the organism which is manifested by differential temperature in the skin. This is a dynamic, not static, process, and as such the clinician must be careful to obtain thermography when the individual is experiencing pain. By the same token, thermography is a useful test to validate the efficacy of sympathetic nerve blocks, nerve root blocks, and facet blocks.

It is also important, as Wexler[6] states, to recognize the limitations of thermography. Just as the thermogram can demonstrate evidence of abnormalities which may be present, it can also demonstrate by an objective means the lack of correlation of thermographic findings with clinical complaints. Unfortunately, there seem to be many more false negatives with thermography as well as other tests than there are false positives. However, one technique for interpreting thermographs that is quite useful is the utilization of comparison of subjectively painful areas with concomitant areas of the body in which the patient reports no pain. The presence of asymmetrical thermography pictures indicates an underlying organic problem, if all artifacts have been eliminated. Thermography is useful in detecting local trauma such as inflammation of a joint, but other types of abnormalities such as primary or secondary bone tumors may produce pain, yet give a normal thermogram. The best bit of advice that Wexler offers is a common-sense consideration: if there is any question regarding the significance of thermography, repeat the finding on a different day.

Wexler[6] also indicates that low back thermographic patterns by themselves have been found to have a 75% accuracy rate when predicting the absence or presence of herniated disc which has been confirmed by surgery. In the same studies, quoted by Wexler, the myelogram was able to predict the presence or absence of herniated disc 84% of the time.

When abnormal thermographies were combined with myelographic findings, the accuracy of prediction was raised to 90%, in surgically confirmed cases.

When patients complained of low back pain associated with radicular pain radiating into one limb, thermography was 93% accurate in predicting the presence or absence of underlying pathology, compared to an 82% accuracy rate for EMG findings. There was a 77% direct correlation between the EMG and the thermography results in the study quoted by Wexler,[6] and he concluded that the accuracy of thermography is comparable to the EMG and to the myelogram. Certainly, when used in conjunction with these two techniques, it further enhances the diagnostic alternatives of the physician.

In a review of 850 articles, Beecher[7] found that pain was a subjective experience and virtually impossible to measure. Therefore, when confronted with a patient complaining of pain, it is imperative that the physician give the patient the benefit of the doubt. Thermography provides a useful tool for detecting a variety of easily overlooked disorders, and is especially useful when these syndromes do not show abnormal findings on x-ray study, EMG, nerve conduction velocity studies, and myelography. While nothing substitutes for a detailed history and physical examination and the use of clinical judgment, thermography, like any useful diagnostic test, does facilitate the confirmation of the clinically diagnosed syndrome.

REFERENCES

1. Merlinger RE: The technique and recording of thermography, in Uematus, S (ed): *Medical Thermography: Theory And Clinical Applications.* Los Angeles, Brentwood Publishing Corp, 1976.
2. Pochaczevsky R: Liquid crystal thermography of the spine and extremities: Its value in the diagnosis of spinal root syndrome. Presented at the Postgraduate Course in Neuroradiology, Columbia-Presbyterian Medical Center, New York May 9-13, 1981.
3. Hendler N, Uematsu S, Long D: Thermographic validation of physical complaints in "psychogenic pain" patients. *Psychosomatics* 1982;23:283–287.
4. Uematsu S, Hendler N, Hungerford D, et al: Thermography and electromyography in the differential diagnosis of chronic back pain syndrome and reflex sympathetic dystrophy. *Electromyog Clin Neurophysiol* 1981, vol 21, pp 165–182.
5. Friedman A, Wood EH: Thermography in vascular headache in Uematsu, S (ed): *Medical Thermography: Theory And Clinical Applications.* Los Angeles, Brentwood Publishing Corp, 1976, pp 80–84.
6. Wexler CE: *An Overview of Liquid Crystal and Electric Lumbar Thoracic and Cervical Thermography.* Tarzana, CA, Thermographic Services Inc, 1981.
7. Beecher HK: Review of pain. *Pharmacol Rev* 1957;9:59–97.

SECTION III
Treatments (Organic)

8 Transcutaneous Electrical Stimulation for Pain: Efficacy and Mechanism of Action

James N. Campbell
Donlin M. Long

Patients with chronic pain have long represented an onerous burden to the medical profession. Pain, although an essential sensory modality, all too frequently persists as a symptom of an underlying uncorrectable disease process, and becomes a disease in its own right. When the cause of pain cannot be treated, the means to obtain pain relief have traditionally been limited to analgesic medication, destructive operative procedures, and indirect measures such as physical therapy. These techniques have serious limitations and frequently aggravate the original pain. The lack of therapeutic options is compounded by the lack of means to assess objectively the presence and severity of the pain. It is unlikely that satisfactory solutions will ever be forthcoming until quantification of clinical pain is possible.

Despite this, progress has been made in the development of novel and effective alternatives in pain treatment, as is testified by the existence of this book. One of the major advances and major areas of interest in this field has been the use of electrotherapy for pain control. It has been found that application of electrical current to the diencephalon,[1a] spinal cord, peripheral nerve, or skin may each have a place in the treatment of pain. The easiest and most benign of these procedures involves application of electric current to the skin. Its technique, usefulness, and mechanism of action will be the topic of this chapter.

Origins of Interest in Electrotherapy

Two developments served to stimulate interest in the use of electrotherapy for the treatment of pain, both occurring in the 1960s. The first was the revival of the original and heuristic concept of Henry Head[1,2] put forward and elaborated by Melzack and Wall[3] under the name, the "gate-control theory." According to this hypothesis, activity in the large primary afferents of the somatosensory system, which normally convey pressure and touch sensations, has an inhibitory effect on the noxious information conveyed by small fibers (C- and A-delta fibers). This inhibitory effect was presumed by Melzack and Wall[3] to take place in the dorsal horn of the spinal cord in the region of the substantia gelatinosa.

Not long after this publication there arose in the Western world growing awareness of the Chinese practice of acupuncture. Although skepticism as to the efficacy of this practice prevailed (as it does now) in scientific circles, considerable public pressure mounted to explore what relevance this ancient art might have for Western medicine.

This intermingling of science and folklore served to stimulate the search for alternate means to manage pain. The idea that pain could be controlled by non-noxious stimulation in contiguous and/or remote areas of the somatosensory system became of interest to clinicians, and initiated what has become a surge of research interest.

In 1967, Wall and Sweet[4] reported that electrical stimulation of the infraorbital nerve produced hypesthesia in the region innervated by this nerve. Since the stimulation itself was thought not to be painful, and because the electrical threshold of large fibers is considerably less than that of small fibers, it was thought that these results represented a demonstration of the inhibitory effects of large fiber primary afferent stimulation on pain perception. The gate-control hypothesis is no longer tenable in its original form, and whether this experiment, in fact, is demonstration of pain reduction by large fiber stimulation will be discussed later in this chapter. Nevertheless, the pioneering findings of Wall and Sweet[4] encouraged the application of electrical stimulation to the peripheral nerves of patients with chronic pain. The first implantable spinal cord stimulators were employed by Shealy as early as 1967, and the first implantable peripheral nerve stimulators were utilized by Long in 1969. The early results of transcutaneous stimulation, and the use of implantable stimulating devices for chronic pain by Wall and Sweet, and Shealy and Long, were promising enough that a number of others have taken up these techniques, and neural modulation is now a major mode of therapy for patients with chronic pain.

History

The analgesic effect of electricity applied to the peripheral nervous system was not a discovery of the 1960s but rather dates to antiquity, as has been noted in a scholarly review of this subject by Kane and Taub.[5] According to Kellaway,[6] one of the first accounts of the application of electrotherapy for pain was made by Scribonius Largus, a Roman physician in the first century A.D. In the following passage the use of the electric fish in the treatment of the age old maladies, gout and headache, is described:

> For any type of gout a live black torpedo should, when the pain begins, be placed under the feet. The patient must stand in a moist shore washed by the sea and he should stay like this until his whole foot and leg up to the knee is numb. This takes away present pain, and prevents pain from coming on if it has not already arisen. Headache, even if it is chronic and unbearable, is taken away and remedied forever by a live black torpedo placed on the spot which is in pain, until the pain ceases. As soon as the numbness has been felt the remedy should be removed lest the ability to feel be taken from the part.[6]

It is of interest to note that the "torpedo " referring to the electric ray, is from the Latin, and literally means numbness or stiffness.

A practical application of electrical stimulation awaited the advent of the electric battery. Several reports of successful use of electricity for relieving pain during tooth extraction appeared.[7–9] As noted by Kane and Taub,[5] Althaus,[10] in 1859, described relief of pain from transcutaneous electrical stimulation applied to the peripheral nerve:

> I . . . applied a rapidly interrupted current to Dr R's ulnar nerve, placing one moistened conductor between the olecranon and the internal condyle, while the other conductor was placed in his hand. I began a current of low tension, such as was not powerful enough to produce contraction of the muscle animated by the ulnar nerve. After the current had acted a few minutes, I increased the intensity, so that a strong flexion of the fourth and little finger was produced. The action of this current was at first painful to bear, and the pain continued to increase during the first few minutes of application; but it soon became less, so that I could further increase the intensity of the current, without causing much inconvenience to Dr R, who became again gradually insensible to

> stronger shocks. The intensity of the current was then increased a third, fourth, and fifth time, and every additional increase was felt distinctly and immediately, but after a certain time the pain excited by very severe shocks was comparatively little. At least the normal sensibility of the ulnar nerve was so much diminished, that a current of such high tension was borne without inconvenience by Dr R, as would have been perfectly unendurable in the beginning of the experiment. Besides, Dr R mentioned a sensation of numbness in the fourth and fifth finger, and that he did not feel the board upon which his fingers rested. The intensity of the current was then diminished, and Dr R was now quite insensible of shocks which had caused him much inconvenience previously. After the current had ceased to act, numbness was still perceived by Dr R in his arm for a certain time. It is therefore obvious that a direct reduction of sensibility of the ulnar nerve was accomplished by electricity, but although the intensity of the current was very high and the velocity of the intermittences very considerable, no complete anesthesia of the skin was produced, as the skin of the hand is not only animated by the ulnar, but also by the median and radial nerve.[5]

Althaus stated that relief of pain from neuralgia was obtained with less intense stimulation. These observations, although made over one hundred years ago, are in agreement with those of others today.

Despite early successes, electrotherapy failed to gain wide support, although occasional reports attesting to its beneficial effects continued into the 1900s. For example, Peterson[11] unaware of previous reports of the analgesic effects of transcutaneous electrical stimulation, suggested that this technique may be used to induce local anesthesia during surgery. Thompson et al[12] described the effects of peripheral nerve stimulation of graded intensity on the sensory modalities subserved by the stimulated nerve. Using a rapidly alternating current with monopolar stimulation applied transcutaneously to the peripheral nerve, it was observed that the thresholds to touch and pressure were most susceptible to electrical stimulation, followed by pain, cold, and heat, in that order.

From this brief historical review it is clear that the idea of using electrical stimulation for control of both acute and chronic pain is an old one. Until most recently, this technique never gained wide acceptance, however, and the reasons for this were probably many. First, the original stimulators were large and awkward to use. Control over stimulus parameters was very limited, as was the availability of the stimulating devices. The control of pain with electrical stimulation never lasted very long, and control of chronic pain depended on frequent visits to the electrotherapist. Second, the emergence of pharmacological techniques for controlling pain lessened the need for electrical analgesia. It is likely, also, that people in the early part of this century and before were less inclined to bring complaints of chronic pain to their physician on a persistent basis. People today expect not to suffer from chronic pain, and this is reflected in the high incidence of operations for pain. The need for more effective means to control pain has evolved as a phenomenon of our generation, paralleling the advance in standards of medical care in general.

Hardware and Techniques

The usefulness of transcutaneous electrical stimulation (TES) of peripheral nerves for the management of chronic pain came as a surprise to the initial users of this technique. Originally developed in an attempt to provide a means of screening patients in order to predict a favorable response to spinal cord stimulation, it soon became apparent that excellent pain relief with TES alone occurred in a small but significant number of patients.[13,14] Sweet and his associates carried out investigations using the stimulators that were utilized commonly in neurophysiological research.[15] Shealy[14] described the usefulness of a simple commercial device available on the open market, the "Electreat." This device consisted of an induction coil which delivered a spike pulse. It was equipped with a crude control for strength of current. Long and Hagfors[13] introduced the first transcutaneous stimulator especially designed for treatment of pain. This initial device was battery operated and employed a variable rectangular wave form with controllable current parameters.

Portable stimulating units, now provided by several companies, differ little in design and stimulus parameters. They are all battery operated and generally produce a spike or a rectangular waveform with variable frequency, voltage, and pulse width control.

Bipolar stimulation is delivered to the skin either directly overlying the area of pain or to the nerve which innervates the painful area. Each electrode should be greater than 4 cm^2 in size in order to minimize skin irritation. The electrodes should be flexible in order that they may be applied uniformly to the skin.[16] Most commercially available electrodes for this purpose are now made of silicone rubber imbedded with carbon particles. The electrodes are coated with a conductive jelly prior to application to the skin. Most units allow for manipulation of repetition, rate, power, and pulse width. These parameters may be adjusted on an empirical basis by both the physician and patient to provide maximal pain relief. Current outputs range from 0 to 70 mA, with voltage up to 90 V. Generally, the repetition rate may be varied from 5 to 200 Hz, while the pulse width can be varied from 50 μsec to several msec.[13]

The stimulus parameters used by patients who achieve excellent pain relief with TES were assessed by Linzer and Long[17] in a group of 14 patients. They found that current requirements ranged from 10 to 70 mA, which corresponds to a current density ranging from 0.5 to 8.5 mA/in^2. The charge per pulse was generally in a range from 1 to 3 μA/sec. Over 70% of the patients found best results with a pulse width ranging from 50 to 100 μsec. Repetition rate in over 80% of the patients was found to be most effective in a range from 10 to 60 Hz.

There are many ways to employ TES in the treatment of patients. Several basic principles must be observed. The patients must be carefully instructed in the use of the technique, and carefully observed so that problems which occur may be solved for them. The position of the electrodes and the parameters of stimulation used may be critical to successful use of TES, and must be carefully evaluated for each patient. The best results in chronic pain have been obtained when initial trials of TES are administered on hospitalized patients, which allows for careful patient instruction. Utilization by outpatients is feasible as long as the patients receive adequate evaluation and instruction in the use of the device. Facilities for the continued evaluation of the patients, monitoring of problems, and maintenance of the stimulating equipment must be available to obtain maximum benefits. At The Johns Hopkins Medical Institutions Pain Treatment Center, TES is one of the first therapeutic modalities offered to patients. It is safe, without major side effects, and does not interfere with diagnostic evaluation or the implementation of a comprehensive pain treatment program.

The procedures for applying TES are simple, and specially trained nurses or technicians are amply qualified to instruct patients in the use of these devices. It is important to distinguish between several categories of patients when attempting to assess the use of TES. In acute pain, such as that following a surgical procedure, the device is primarily employed by specially trained personnel to provide pain relief over a short period of time. The same is true of pains which may be classified as less serious or minor, for instance, athletic injuries, the acute low back or cervical syndromes, and minor soft tissue trauma. Chronic pain represents the greatest therapeutic challenge, and patients with chronic pain require a much longer period of time for evaluation and treatment if TES is to achieve optimal results.

The following principles have emerged from practical experience with over 1000 patients.

1. Electrodes may be placed in the region overlying a painful area (on occasion, this worsens pain, and the electrodes must be moved proximal to the pain) or over a major nerve which innervates the painful area.
2. Stimulation applied distal to the origin of pain almost never gives rise to satisfactory long-term benefits and sometimes aggravates the pain. Most patients who achieve effective pain relief feel tingling or some other sensation in the painful area when TES is applied.

3. Stimulating units should provide patients with flexible control of voltage, pulse width, and repetition rate, since the ideal stimulus parameters vary from patient to patient. However, the range is relatively narrow for optimum results, and it is also important to be certain that patients have explored the parameter areas most likely to give good pain control.
4. Stimulating units should be small so that they may be easily and inconspicuously carried. Application of electrodes and design of the device must allow the patient to undertake his usual daily activities while TES is being applied.
5. Patients who initially state that stimulation is ineffective will rarely achieve suitable pain relief with electrodes remaining in the same location. Before making this decision, a several-hour trial of stimulation is warranted. Failure of relief, when electrodes are in a location such that TES does not evoke paresthesias referred to the painful region, has no bearing on eventual success.
6. TES does not offer a cure for pain. Successful use of the technique is palliative, and does not replace the need for accurate diagnosis. Pain relief which lasts more than a few hours after termination of stimulation may be related to other factors such as muscular relaxation, humoral effect, psychogenic overlay, or the natural course of the pain.
7. Patients who have an initial favorable response to TES require at least several weeks to determine whether the technique is to have a lasting value. The patient should be free to rent a stimulating device for a variable length of time before the decision to purchase one is made by the patient and physician.
8. Patients require continued instruction with these devices and assistance with proper purchase. It is very important that this instruction be readily available for them if the results of therapy are to be maximized.
9. Patients who are first introduced to TES in the setting of a pain treatment center frequently have a favorable response which is not maintained during subsequent trials. This early success most likely represents a placebo response, and rarely lasts more than 48 hours. Most patients, attaining good relief of pain at the end of one month, continue to achieve this pain relief and continue to use the device on a long-term basis.

Pattern of Use

In Figure 8-1 the location site of electrodes used to treat chronic pain in four different patients is illustrated. These areas of stimulation may be varied somewhat to avoid skin irritation to any one area.

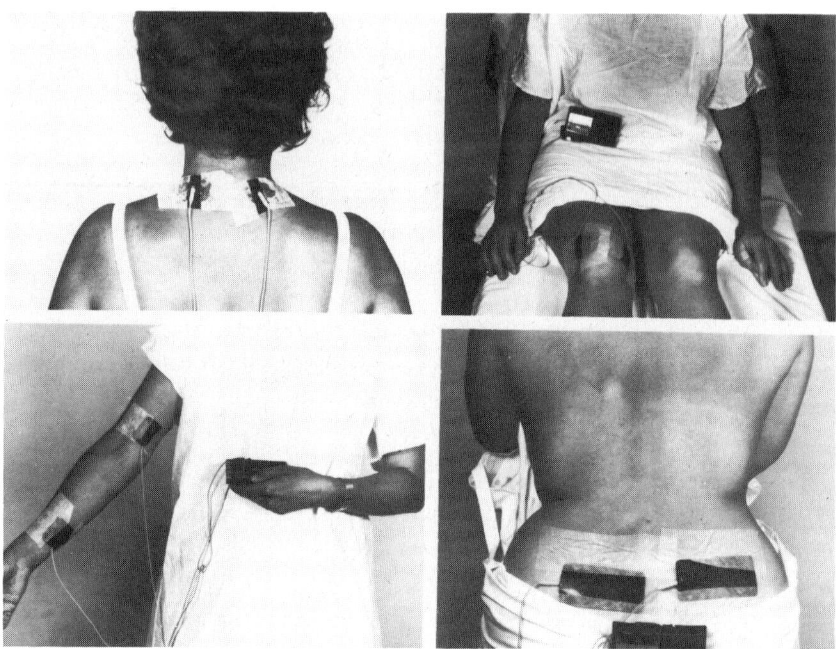

Figure 8-1 Four different patients are shown using transcutaneous nerve stimulation. From left to right, beginning with the top row, the conditions being treated are whiplash injury to the cervical spine, arthritis of the knee, ulnar nerve distribution pain due to ulnar nerve injury, and lumbar pain following unsuccessful lumbar disc surgery.

The length of time of stimulation and frequency of use varies considerably from patient to patient. The type of pain which the patient has is important in determining the pattern of use of the device. Patients with minor pain such as that accompanying chronic low back ailments or the cervical syndrome may often obtain pain relief with less than an hour of use. This relief characteristically will persist for a long period of time. Patients with acute pain such as that seen in the postoperative period utilize TES for longer periods of time, but often will not require continuous stimulation. Stimulation of the operative site for one to two hours out of each four- to six-hour period may give substantial pain relief. Patients with severe chronic pain typically use the device 8 to 16 hours per day. It is important that the electrodes be coated evenly with electrode jelly to minimize skin irritation and discomfort. The electrodes should be removed for at least eight hours per day to further minimize skin irritation.

Clinical Efficacy

There is now a large body of evidence which confirms a role for the use of TES in the treatment of pain. We shall now consider the scope of this role and expectations for successful use of this technique.

It is inherently unsatisfactory to be able only to treat the symptom of a disease and not be able to correct the cause. Transcutaneous electrical stimulation is a technique to which the physician may resort to provide the patient with symptomatic relief and not one which will offer definitive treatment. Unlike other therapeutic options for the patient in chronic pain, however, TES is quite free from danger to the patient. The technique has no addictive potential and has little in the way of adverse side effects. Unlike neurosurgical ablative procedures, there is no threat of disruption of normal neurological function. It is easy to implement; if it fails to work little is lost.

Depending on the patient population, anywhere from 10% to 35% of patients suffering from otherwise intractable pain will achieve long-term excellent pain relief from use of TES.[18,19] The criteria for an excellent result vary from study to study, but at a minimum this means that a patient previously incapacitated with pain is able to obtain nearly complete relief from pain during this period. Between 30% and 50% of patients with chronic pain find TES to be a useful adjunct to other forms of pain therapy on a long-term basis.

The success of TES treatment in part depends on the origin of the pain. Patients with peripheral neuropathy, pain of central origin, and those with pain presumed to be secondary to psychogenic factors almost never achieve satisfactory pain relief using this technique. Patients with postherpetic neuralgia, phantom limb pain, stump pain, branchial plexus injury, peripheral nerve trauma, and arthritis are most consistently helped with TES. In a series of 39 patients with one of these diagnoses reported by Long and Hagfors,[13] 70% of the patients obtained excellent pain relief using TES on a long-term basis. Patients with chronic low back pain or cervical spine pain, with or without radiculopathy, constitute the majority of patients with chronic pain in most pain centers. In a group of 301 such patients, approximately 30% of the patients obtained excellent pain relief with TES. Patients with reflex sympathetic dystrophy or causalgia may have benefit if treated early in the context of their disorder.[20]

In addition to chronic pain, TES may have a role in the treatment of acute pain. Hymes and his associates[21] first called attention to the fact that postoperative pain could be greatly alleviated by the use of TES. First, in a retrospective study and then in a prospective fashion, these authors discovered that patients undergoing thoracotomy and laparotomy were significantly improved when TES was employed in the postoperative period. The need for narcotics was reduced and postoperative problems with atelectasis and ileus were considerably lessened. Van der Ark and McGrath[22] found that 77% of patients receiving TES for pain following thoracic and abdominal surgical procedures had substantial reduction in pain, as manifested by a reduction in verbal ratings of pain, and a reduction or elimination of narcotic intake. The usefulness of TES for control of pain resulting from such things as orthopedic injuries is limited in nonhospitalized patients by the cost and availability of stimulating units. The technique is quite useful in hospitalized patients and may reduce the need for analgesic medications. However, until it is as easy for the physician to order TES as it is to write an order for narcotics, it is unlikely that the technique will find widespread use in the hospital setting.

Mechanism of Action

Several hypotheses have been proposed to explain how TES relieves pain. These ideas may be divided into those in which direct effects on the peripheral nerve fibers themselves are postulated, and those in which it is proposed that TES modifies the transmission of nociceptive information in the central nervous system (CNS).

In the first proposal, it is postulated that the application of electrical current to the peripheral nerve at a location interposed between the source of the pain and the spinal cord induces an axonal blockade of activity in the primary afferent nociceptive fibers, and thereby prevents pain perception. The evidence that this mechanism plays at least some role in reducing pain during TES is considerable.

To understand better the effects of TES on normal pain perception, Campbell and Taub[23] studied the electrical parameters and stimulus locations necessary to alter normal pain perception. It was found that at levels of electrical stimulation necessary to induce cutaneous analgesia, there was loss of the A-delta elevation in the compound action potential recording. Effects on pain threshold were found only at points distal to the point of stimulation. It was further observed that stimulus frequencies greater than 10 Hz were necessary to obtain cutaneous analgesia. The electrical stimuli were not in themselves painful unless introduced suddenly, several minutes after any prior stimulation. The pain resulting in this instance was brief, lasting a matter of seconds. These data were taken as evidence that electrical analgesia resulting from TES in normal subjects was due at least in part to an axonal blockade occurring in the primary afferent nociceptive fibers.

It was also postulated that a momentary activation of nociceptive fibers (which must precede axonal blockade) dispersed over time in patients with preexisting pain in the area innervated by the activated neurons may not be perceived. Thus, TES for clinical pain would not necessarily be expected to be even momentarily painful, despite the initial activation of nociceptive fibers prior to axonal blockade.

Corroboration of This Hypothesis

Further evidence for these ideas was presented by Ignelzi and Nyquist.[24] In this experiment, the effects of peripheral nerve stimulation on the compound action potential elicited by a subsequent supramaximal electric shock were studied in the cat. It was found that stimulation with electrical parameters similar to those used clinically to establish pain relief in humans led to a reduction in the height of the A-delta wave in the compound action potential recording. An example of these findings is shown in Figure 8-2. The first wave represents the A-beta wave adjacent to the electrical artifact. The second elevation is the A-delta wave. It is apparent that the degree of blockade of A-delta and A-beta units varies directly with the length of the conditioning stimulus. The degree of blockade is also increased by an increase in the voltage of stimulation. As found by Campbell and Taub,[23] blockade is antedated by an increase in conduction time.

It is possible that the reduction of the A-delta portion of the compound action potential in these two experiments merely represents a dispersion of the latencies of the single A-delta units, and therefore does not represent a conduction block. In addition, recording techniques did not allow identification of the wave associated with C-fiber activation. It is thus desirable to study the effects of electrical stimulation on individual A-delta and C units. This was accomplished by Torebjörk and Hallin[25] in human subjects.

Single units thought to subserve nociception which had conduction velocities in the C-fiber range were recorded from microelectrodes inserted percutaneously into peripheral nerves of unanesthetized human subjects. These units could be activated with electric shocks applied through intradermal electrodes placed near the receptive field of the respective C-fibers. Trains of electric shocks with a pulse width of 50 to 100 μsec were delivered through the electrode. The response latency of these units increased as the stimulus frequency was increased from 0.5 to

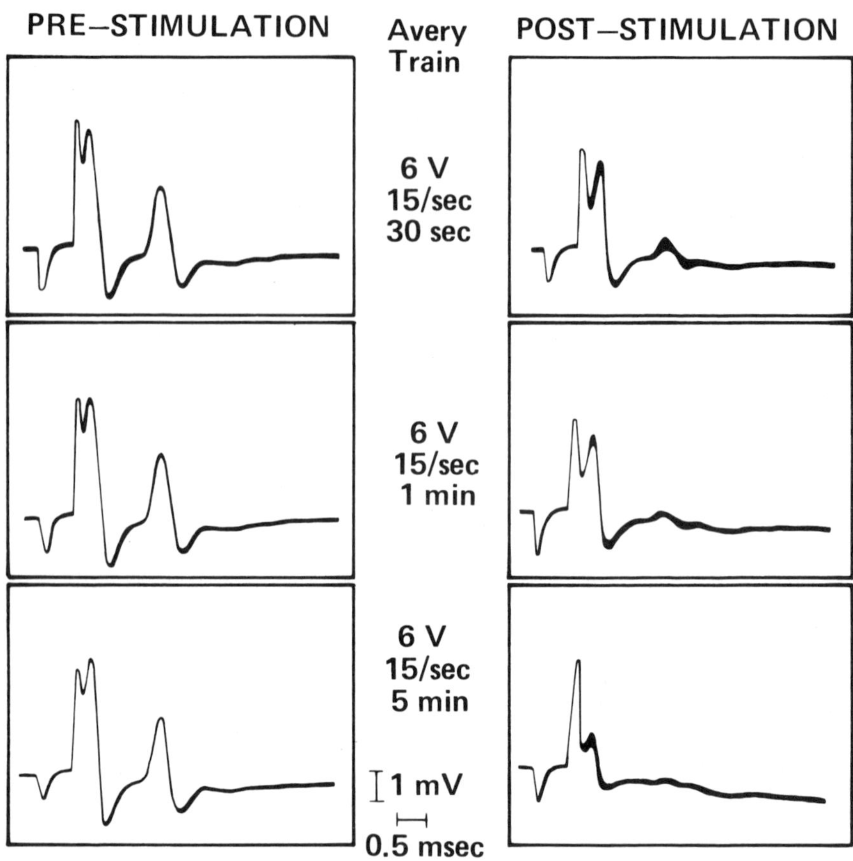

Figure 8-2 The effects of peripheral nerve stimulation on the A-delta component of the compound action potential. The compound action potential before and after a 30 sec, 1 min, and 5 min 6 volt 15/sec train of stimuli is shown. As the stimulus train is increased in duration, the A-delta wave becomes progressively smaller (from Ignelzi and Nyquist,[24] with permission).

10 Hz. At frequencies of 10 Hz pronounced blocking occurred. This was accompanied by loss of pain from the introduced shock and an elevation of pain threshold tested with pinprick stimuli. The recovery from such blocking was not systematically investigated, but the effect was still notable after 30 sec of rest from electrical stimulation. In the larger myelinated fibers, blocking and decreases in conduction velocity also occurred but required stimulus frequencies from 50 to 100 Hz. It is of interest to note in the report of Linzer and Long[16] that patients who had excellent pain relief with TES generally preferred stimulus frequencies between 10 to 60 Hz. Such frequencies may be expected to have a preferential blocking effect on small fibers and, therefore, reduce pain sensation.

Further corroboration of this hypothesis was presented by Wall and Gutnick[26] in an electrophysiological study of experimentally produced neuromas in rats. It was shown that a 100 Hz, six-second train of bipolar electrical stimulation applied to the peripheral nerve led to a marked increase of the electrical threshold, and loss of spontaneous activity in A-delta fibers which were presumed to innervate the neuroma (techniques did not allow for C-fiber recordings). This change in excitability lasted anywhere from minutes to as long as one hour. This contrasted with a more prompt return to normal in A-delta units which innervated histologically normal areas. The results of this experiment suggest, therefore, that pain arising from neuromas may be more susceptible to the blocking effects of TES than other types of pain. This conclusion is in agreement with studies in human patients with implanted peripheral nerve stimulators in which it has been found that chronic pain from peripheral nerve trauma responds most satisfactorily to stimulation.[27]

The phenomenon of frequency dependent conduction block of axons described here is analogous to the phenomenon of "Wedensky inhibition" originally described in 1903. Working with nerve-muscle preparations, Wedensky[28] found that a stimulus strong enough to elicit a contraction may fail to stimulate when it is repeated at certain relatively rapid rates. It has subsequently been demonstrated with single unit recordings that this results from a localized conduction block, ie, block of the propagation of the action potential in the axon.

Much has been learned recently regarding the mechanism and requirements of frequency related conduction block. The question has attracted additional interest because of evidence which suggests that conduction block may occur as a part of normal neuronal activity. For example, it has been shown that points of axonal branching and areas with increasing fiber diameter are especially vulnerable to frequency related conduction block.[29-33]

Theoretical and experimental evidence collected by several authors suggests that this phenomenon may be related to an increased concentration of potassium in the space outside the axolemma during repetitive firing of an axon.[34-38] From the Nernst equation it would be predicted that such a change would result in membrane depolarization. Inactivation of sodium conductance occurs both with increases in external potassium concentration and prolonged depolarization. Because sodium conductance is necessary for propagation of the action potential, these changes may lead to a conduction block. Adelman and Fitzhugh[34] modified the Hodgkin and Huxley equations to take into consideration changes in K^+ concentration during repetitive firing. They were able to predict and experimentally verify conduction block from repetitive firing of the squid giant axon using the modified equations. In addition the changes in spike amplitude and response latency observed prior to block were predicted from these equations.

It is predicted that factors in the environment of the axon which impede the diffusion of potassium from the axon will increase the susceptibility to frequency related conduction block. Smith and Hatt[39] demonstrated in the crayfish that an area of motor axon which passes through dense connective tissue was very susceptible to blockade with repetitive stimulation. Because the axon has no geometrical variation in this region, it was concluded by the authors that the dense connective tissue surrounding the axon acted as a barrier to the diffusion of potassium and may, therefore, account for the observed conduction block. Regardless of the mechanism, the importance of such things as connective tissue surrounding the axon in increasing the susceptibility to conduction block invites speculation that similar mechanism explains the susceptibility to conduction block of fibers which innervate neuromas (see previous discussion of experiment by Wall and Gutnick[26]).

Torebjörk and Hallin[25] have shown that C fibers are more susceptible to conduction block than the large myelinated fibers. This too can be explained in terms of the environment of the axon. Ruch and Patton[40] have stated that "the immediate extracellular space of the C fiber is peculiarly restricted in such a way that extracellular accumulation of potassium may well occur during repetitive activity." Thus, frequency related conduction block would be predicted to be more prominent in C fibers.

One final observation deserves mention. It has been observed that TES may relieve chronic pain without any other easily demonstrable effect on sensation. This observation has in the past posed difficulties for those who proposed that a peripheral axonal blockade of nociceptive afferents was important in producing TES-related analgesia. Because injured nerves are surrounded by increased amounts of connective tissue, it would be predicted that these fibers would be most susceptible to frequency related conduction block. It is, therefore, understandable how TES might alleviate pathological pain without interfering with other functions subserved by the stimulated peripheral nerve.

It deserves to be emphasized that in order for frequency related conduction block to occur, the fiber in question, in this case the A-delta and/or C fiber, must be initially activated before conduction block can occur. It remains to be demonstrated that C fibers may be activated using the electrical parameters utilized during TES. Until this is demonstrated the "frequency related conduction block hypothesis" must be regarded to be tentative, though there is circumstantial evidence to support it.

Anodal and Cathodal Blockade

A special type of axonal conduction block may be induced with DC currents of electricity. These have been termed cathodal and anodal block. Induction of a cathodal block requires that a subthreshold depolarizing current be applied. Although there is an initial increase in excitability, a prolonged subthreshold stimulus may reduce sodium conductance to the point that a stronger than normal stimulus is required to activate the axon in this region. Induction of an anodal blockade requires that a hyperpolarizing current be applied. The potential shift required to reach threshold for activation is thereby increased.

These types of block are clearly different from those proposed to occur during TES. Anodal blockade has been used to produce local anesthesia in patients undergoing dental procedures.[41–44] For example, anodal current may be applied through the drill to the tooth pulp during restorations. The safety of this procedure has not yet been fully established, although commercial devices for utilizing this procedure are apparently available in the Soviet Union.[45] Unlike TES, this procedure blocks activity in the large fibers prior to including a conduction block in C fibers.[46] The electrical parameters are much different than those used in TES. Anodal block requires monopolar stimulation with a continuous DC current. TES, in contrast, involves bipolar stimulation with rapidly applied stimuli with brief pulse widths. It is, therefore, quite unlikely that either a cathodal or anodal block occurs during the type of TES under discussion in this chapter.

The Role of Central Mechanism

Not all sensory information entering the CNS from peripheral nerve fibers is perceived. There exists, therefore, control systems within the CNS that determine which and how much sensory information shall reach consciousness. Nociceptive information maintains a high priority in sensory experience as is commensurate with the importance of such information in minimizing harm to the organism from damaging stimuli. It has been postulated that TES may activate normally present CNS control systems, and thereby suppress the transmission of nociceptive information to CNS areas which subserve the sensation of pain and its affective attributes.

Just how such control systems may work, and what relevance known control systems may have in explaining the effects of TES has invited a surfeit of speculation. Certain ideas may be discounted, however. First is the idea that TES works by diverting attention from the pain. The fact that the stimulation must be applied to the nerve which transmits the nociceptive signal, and that when applied to an area remote to this nerve has no effect reduces the possibility that perceptual diversion plays an important role.

It has been popular to attribute the effects of TES-induced analgesia to an inhibitory effect of large primary afferent fiber activity on centrally located neurons, which is associated with pain perception. Two experimental approaches have been used to study this possibility. In the first approach, the effects of peripheral nerve stimulation on pain perception in the region innervated by that nerve were studied in human subjects. When Wall and Sweet[4] did this, they observed hypalgesia with levels of stimulation which were in themselves not painful. They concluded from this that the hypalgesia resulted from selective large-fiber stimulation. It has already been noted, however, that when electrophysiological measurements of the effects of such stimulation are made, there is evidence for inactivation of the primary afferent nociceptive fibers.[23,24] Nathan and Rudge[47] also found that stimulation of large primary fibers in itself had no effect on either pain threshold or pain tolerance in normal human subjects.

In the second approach, the effects of large-fiber stimulation may be studied in terms of their effects on central neurons, activity of which is associated with the perception of pain. This experiment is presently difficult to conduct because of uncertainties in regard to which central neurons subserve nociception.

The activity of spinothalamic neurons in response to C-fiber volleys as a function of the presence or absence of coincident A-fiber volleys has been studied. Price and Wagman[48] found in monkeys that central inhibition and facilitation can result from maximal stimulation of either A or C fibers without necessity of interaction between effects of these two groups. Manfredi[49] found that A- and C-fiber volleys had only an additive effect on the contralateral (and ipsilateral) anterolateral potential (presumed to be an index of activity in the spinothalamic tract) in the cat.

Nociceptive cells of the lamina I in the anesthetized cat have been described in which response to noxious cutaneous stimuli may be suppressed by such things as hair movement in the receptive field.[50] Peripheral nerve stimulation was also reported to suppress the response of lamina I nociceptive units.[51] There was a positive correlation between the amount of suppression and the intensity of electrical stimulation delivered to the peripheral nerve, but data were not provided by which it could be reliably determined whether large-fiber activation by itself could suppress the response of these nociceptive units. No such interaction has been demonstrated in the primate. This, in combination with the lack of notable effects of large-fiber activation on the subjective magnitude of pain judged by human subjects, reduces the possibility that such a central interaction is of much importance in normal pain perception, at least in humans.

The possibility that large fiber stimulation may affect higher order nociceptive neurons has been largely unexplored. This is recent evidence that a descending control system exists in the dorsolateral funiculus of the spinal cord, which may mediate pain relief elicited by periaqueductal and pretectal stimulation.[52] In a study of rats,[53] it was found that bilateral sectioning of the dorsolateral funiculus blocked morphine-induced analgesia, but had no effect on analgesia produced by transcutaneous stimulation. This suggests that TES does not affect pain perception by way of actions of periaqueductal structures associated with morphine-induced analgesia.

In summary, there is evidence that TES-induced pain relief may be mediated by effects on the peripheral nerve itself. Evidence for centrally mediated effects of TES on pain perception is as yet scanty.

Conclusions

Transcutaneous electrical stimulation is a benign and simple form of therapy which may be effective in relieving pain which fails to respond to conventional therapy. There is a small incidence of skin irritation, and it may be cumbersome for the patient to carry the power supply and attach the electrodes to the skin on a daily basis. Despite this drawback, patients with chronic low back pain (one of the most difficult groups to help with any form of therapy) have a long-term success rate which is striking. In other forms of pain, expectations for success may be even higher. Patients with central pain or pain in which it may be difficult to apply the stimulation to the peripheral nerve proximal to the area from which the pain arises form a group which generally will not receive benefit from TES therapy.

Other techniques in which peripheral nerve stimulators are attached directly to the nerve[27,54] or in which epidural electrodes are placed over posterior roots (DM Long, unpublished data, 1977) offer a means of stimulation in which some of the problems encountered with TES may be overcome. The principal advantage of these techniques is that the stimulation may be applied more directly to the nerve. Problems with skin irritation are largely obviated and the intensity of the stimulus to the nerve is increased. Currently, these devices require an external power supply in order to activate the implanted electrodes. Research is now underway, however, to develop a power supply which may be permanently implanted and periodically recharged from an external source (R Fischell, unpublished data 1977). Such a device would be a great advantage to the patient who required long-term CNS stimulation for relief of pain.

In this chapter the mechanism by which TES relieves pain was considered in some detail. Although conclusions must as yet be tentative, there is evidence to suggest that a blockade of activity in the primary afferent nociceptive fibers plays at least some role in pain reduction. A mechanism by which such a blockade may occur is proposed to involve a rate related conduction block (analogous to "Wedensky inhibition"), which in turn may be due to accumulation of potassium in the periaxonal space surrounding the primary afferent nociceptive fibers. Central mechanisms may also be important in understanding TES-related analgesia, but evidence at this time is sparse.

Whatever the mechanism, TES appears to be a valid way of treating many patients previously incapacitated by otherwise intractable chronic pain. It is safe, relatively inexpensive, and effective over long periods of time for many of these patients.

REFERENCES

1a. Limoge A: *An Introduction to Electroanesthesia.* Baltimore, University Park Press, 1975.
1. Head H (in conjunction with WHR Rivers, G Holmes, J Sherren, T Thompson, G Riddock). *Studies in Neurology.* London, Oxford Univ Press, vols 1 and 2, 1920.
2. Hanson RA: Henry Head's work on sensation. *Brain* 1961;84:535–550.
3. Melzack R, Wall PD: Pain mechanisms: A new theory. *Science* 1965;150:971–979.
4. Wall PD, Sweet WH: Temporary abolition of pain in man. *Science* 1967;155:108–109.
5. Kane K, Taub A: A history of local electrical analgesia. *Pain* 1975;1:125–138.
6. Kellaway P: The part played by electric fish in the early history of bioelectricity and electrotherapy. *Bull Hist Med* 1946;20:112–137.
7. Clark FY: Electricity as an anesthetic. *Dent News Letter* 1858;12:75.
8. Francis JB: Extracting teeth by galvinism. *Dent Rep* 1858;9:65–69.
9. Morel-Lavallée UAF: Académie de Médicine: Electrisation appliqué avec un success complet à l'extraction des dents, et oux opérations avec l'instrument tranchant. *Arch Gén Méd* 1859;1:97.
10. Althaus J: *A Treatise on Medical Electricity, Theoretical and Practical, and Its Use in the Treatment of Paralysis, Neuralgia, and Other Diseases.* London, Trubner, 1859 and 1970.
11. Peterson E: Local electrical anesthesia. *Science* 1933;77:326.
12. Thompson IM, Banks GF, Barron A, et al: Differential elevations of cutaneous sensory thresholds by alternating currents applied to a nerve. *Univ Calif Publ Anat* 1934;1:167–194.
13. Long DM Hagfors N: Electrical stimulation in the nervous system: The current status of electrical stimulation of the nervous system for relief of pain. *Pain* 1975;1:109–123.
14. Shealy CN, Transcutaneous electrical stimulation for control of pain. *Clin Neurosurg* 1974;21:269–277.
15. Sweet WH, Wepsic JG: Treatment of chronic pain by stimulation of fibers of primary afferent neurons. *Trans Am Neurol Assoc* 1968;93:103–107.
16. Ray CD, Maurer DD: Electrical neurological stimulation systems: A review of contemporary methodology. *Surg Neurol* 1975;4:82–90.
17. Linzer M, Long DM: Transcutaneous neural stimulation for relief of pain. *IEEE Trans Biomed Eng* 1976;23:341–345.
18. Loeser J, Black R, Christman A: Relief of pain by transcutaneous stimulation. *J Neurosurg* 1975;42:308–314.

19. Long DM, Carolan MT: Cutaneous afferent stimulation in the treatment of chronic pain, in Bonica JJ (ed): *International Symposium on Pain Advances in Neurology*. New York, Raven Press, 1974, vol 4, pp 727–732.
20. Meyer GA, Fields HL: Causalgia treated by selective large fiber stimulation of peripheral nerve. *Brain* 1972;95:163–168.
21. Hymes AC, Roab DE, Yonehira EG, et al: Electrical surface stimulation for the control of acute post-operative pain and prevention of ileus. *Surg Forum* 1973;24:273–276.
22. Van der Ark GD, McGrath K: Transcutaneous electrical stimulation in treatment of postoperative pain. *Am J Surg* 1975;130:338–340.
23. Campbell JN, Taub A: Local analgesia from percutaneous electrical stimulation:A peripheral mechanism. *Arch Neurol* 1973;28:347–350.
24. Ignelzi RJ, Nyquist J: Direct effect of electrical stimulation on peripheral nerve evoked activity: Implications in pain relief. *J Neurosurg* 1976; 45:159–165.
25. Torebjörk HE, Hallin RG: Responses in human A and C fibers to repeated electrical intradermal stimulation. *J Neurol Neurosurg Psychiatry* 1974;37:653–664.
26. Wall PD, Gutnick M: Ongoing activity in peripheral nerves: The physiology and pharmacology of impulses originating from a neuron. *Exp Neurol* 1974;43:580–593.
27. Campbell JN, Long DM: Peripheral nerve stimulation in the treatment of intractable pain. *J Neurosurg* 1976;45:692–699.
28. Wedensky NE: Die Erregung, Hemmung und Narkose. *Pfluegers Arch* 1903;100:1–144.
29. Chung S, Raymond SA, Lettvin JY: Multiple meaning in single visual units. *Brain Behav Evol* 1970;3:72–101.
30. Grossman Y, Spira ME, Parnas I: Differential flow of information into branches of a single axon. *Brain Res* 1973;64:379–386.
31. Parnas I: Differential block at high frequency of branches of a single axon innervating two muscles. *J Neurophysiol* 1972;35:903–914.
32. Taub L, Hughs GM: Modes of initiation and propagation of spikes in the branching axon of the molluscan central neurons. *J Gen Physiol* 1963;46:533–549.
33. Waxman SG: Regional differentiation of the axon: A review with reference to the concept of the multiplex neuron. *Brain Res* 1972;47:269–280.
34. Adelman WJ, Fitzhugh R: Solutions of the Hodgkin-Huxley equations modified for potassium accumulation in a periaxonal space. *Fed Proc* 1975;34:1322–1329.
35. Frankenhaeuser B, Hodgkin AL: The after-effects of impulses in the giant nerve fibers of *Loligo*. *J Physiol* 1956;131:341–376.
36. Adelman WJ, Palti Y: The influence of external potassium on the inactivation of the sodium current in the giant axon of the squid. *J Gen Physiol* 1969;53:685–703.
37. Parnas I, Hochstein S, Parnas H: Theoretical analysis of parameters leading to frequency modulation along an inhomogeneous axon. *J Neurophysiol* 1976;39:909–923.
38. Spira, ME, Yarom, Y, Parnas I: Modulation of spike frequency by regions of special geometry and by synaptic inputs. *J Neurophysiol* 1976;39: 882–899.
39. Smith DD, Hatt H: Axon conduction block in a region of dense connective tissue in crayfish. *J Neurophysiol* 1976;39:794–801.
40. Ruch TC, Patton HD: *Physiology and Biophysics*. Philadelphia, WB Saunders Co, 1966, p 80.

41. Fields RW, Tacke RB, Savara BS: Pulpal anodal blockade of trigeminal field potentials elicited by tooth stimulation in the cat. *Exp Neurol* 1975;47:229–239.
42. Brooks B, Reiss R, Umans R: Local electroanesthesia in dentistry. *J Dent Res* 1970;49:298–300.
43. Douglas BL: Anesthesia by electricity. *NY State Dent J* 1955;21:28–29.
44. Reid KH: Mechanism of action of dental electroanesthesia. *Nature* 1974;247:150–151.
45. Newman PP: Electrical method for controlling pain. *Nature* 1973; 243:474–475.
46. Manfredi M: Differential block of conduction of larger fibers in peripheral nerve by direct current. *Arch Ital Biol* 1970;108:52–71.
47. Nathan PW, Rudge P: Testing the gate-control theory of pain in man. *J Neurol Neurosurg Psychiatry* 1974;37:1366–1372.
48. Price DD, Wagman IH: Physiological roles of A and C fiber inputs to the spinal dorsal horn of *Macacca Mulatta. Exp Neurol* 1970;29:383–399.
49. Manfredi M: Modulation of sensory projections in anterolateral column of cat spinal cord by peripheral afferents of different size. *Arch Ital Biol* 1970;108:72–105.
50. Iggo A: Activation of cutaneous nociceptors and their actions on dorsal horn neurones, in Bonica JJ (ed): *Pain, Advances in Neurology.* New York, Raven Press, 1974, vol 4, pp 1–9.
51. Cervero F, Iggo A, Ogawa H: Nociceptor-driven dorsal horn neurones in the lumbar spinal cord of the cat. *Pain* 1976;2:5–24.
52. Mayer DJ, Price DD: Central nervous system mechanisms of analgesia. *Pain* 1976;2:379–404.
53. Price DD, Hayes RL, Bennett GJ, et al: Effects of dorsolateral spinal cord lesions on narcotic and non-narcotic analgesia in the rat. Presented at the Sixth Annual Meeting of the Society for Neuroscience, Toronto, 1976.
54. Long DM: Electrical stimulation for relief of pain from chronic nerve injury. *J Neurosurg* 1973;39:718–722.

9 Sphenopalatine Ganglion Block in Treatment of Acute and Chronic Pain

Milton A. Reder
Alan S. Hymanson
Milton Reder

In recent years there has been a resurgence of interest in topical anesthetization of the sphenopalatine (nasal) ganglion, an outpatient procedure originally described many years ago, for the treatment of a variety of acute and chronic pain syndromes. Researchers at several major centers and numerous private practitioners are actively investigating the wide ranging uses of this technique, with highly encouraging results.

Anatomy

The sphenopalatine ganglion (alternately called pterygopalatine, nasal, or Meckel's ganglion) is one of the four autonomic ganglia in the head as shown in Figure 9-1, which illustrates the gross anatomy of the area. The ganglion is located in the pterygopalatine fossa, posterior to the middle turbinate, and is covered by a 1- to 5-mm layer of connective tissue and mucous membrane. This places it within diffusing distance of a topically applied anesthetic. The ganglion is a 5-mm triangular structure and is the largest collection of neurons in the head outside of the brain itself. There are major branches from the

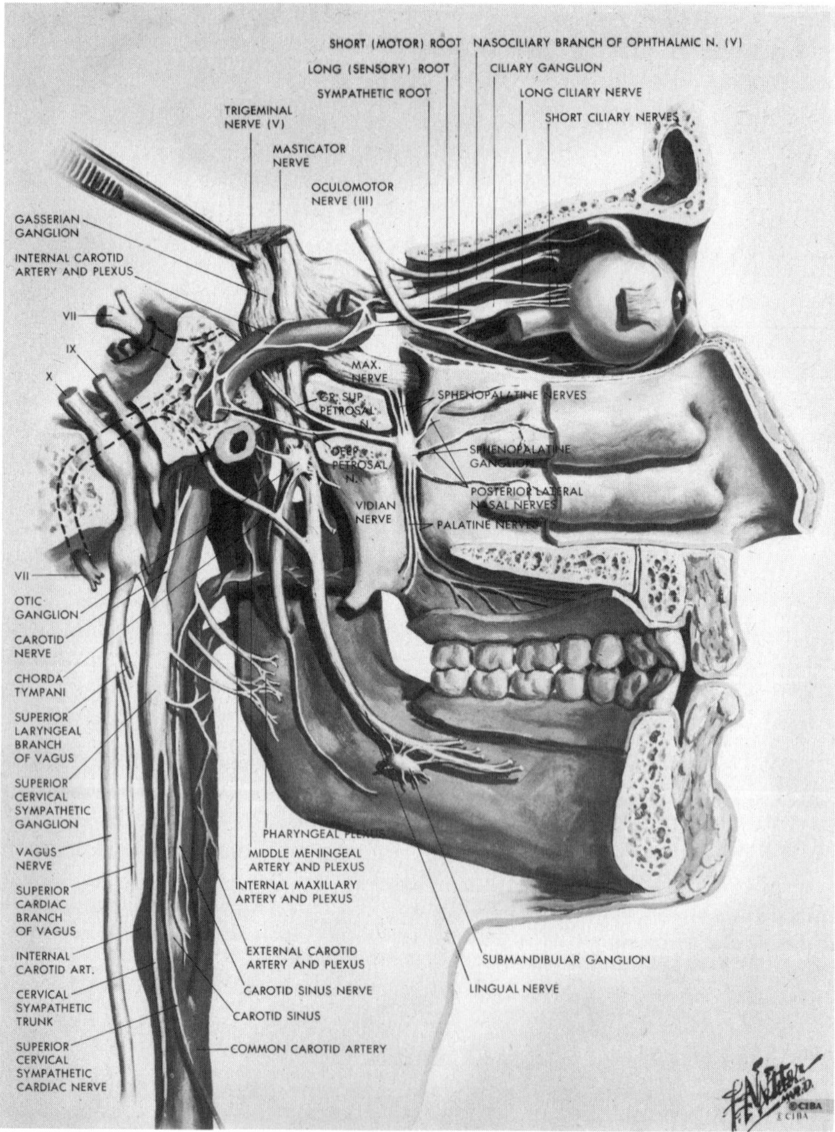

Figure 9-1 Autonomic nerves in the head. ©Copyright 1953, 1972, CIBA Pharmaceutical Company, Division of CIBA-GEIGY Corporation. Reprinted with permission from *The CIBA Collection of Medical Illustrations* illustrated by Frank H. Netter, MD. All rights reserved.

sphenopalatine ganglion to the trigeminal nerve, facial nerve, and carotid plexus, the latter providing a direct communication with the superior cervical sympathetic ganglion.

Functional Considerations

From a physiologic standpoint, Figure 9-2 shows the neuronal wiring diagram of the sphenopalatine ganglion. Functionally, there are three routes of the sphenopalatine ganglion: sensory, visceral motor (or parasympathetic), and sympathetic. Anatomically, there is overlap between these routes, but in simplest terms the sensory root is typified by the connection with the maxillary division of the trigeminal nerve. This area consists of fibers with cell bodies located in the trigeminal ganglion. They are afferent neurons which synapse in the central nervous system on substantia gelatinosa and other cells of the sensory nucleus of V in the pons, relaying to the ventroposteromedial thalamic nucleus. The pain fibers included here have a high rate of spontaneous activity, and it has

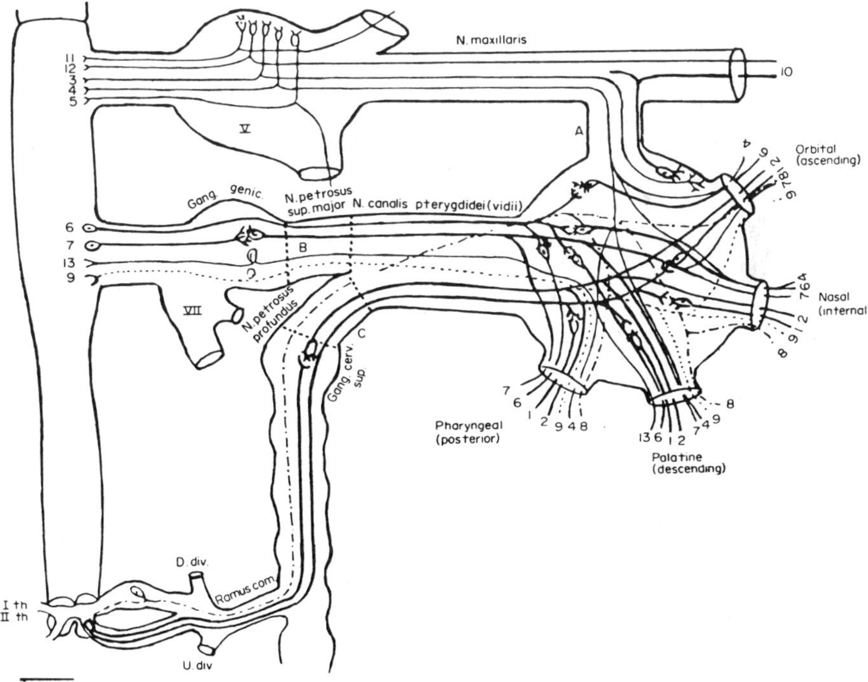

Figure 9-2 Connections of the sphenopalatine ganglion. From Sluder G: The anatomical and clinical relations of the sphenopalatine ganglion to the nose. *NY State J Med* 1909;90:293–298.

been hypothesized that they modulate the rostral transmissions of pain information from the periphery, acting like a gate-control mechanism (see Figure 9-3A). Blockade of the sphenopalatine ganglion may inhibit this baseline tonic activity and in so doing, close the gate, acting through the same mechanism as that proposed to explain the analgesia of transcutaneous nerve stimulation, but at a higher level in the CNS. This connection may explain the success of sphenopalatine ganglion block in tic douloureux.

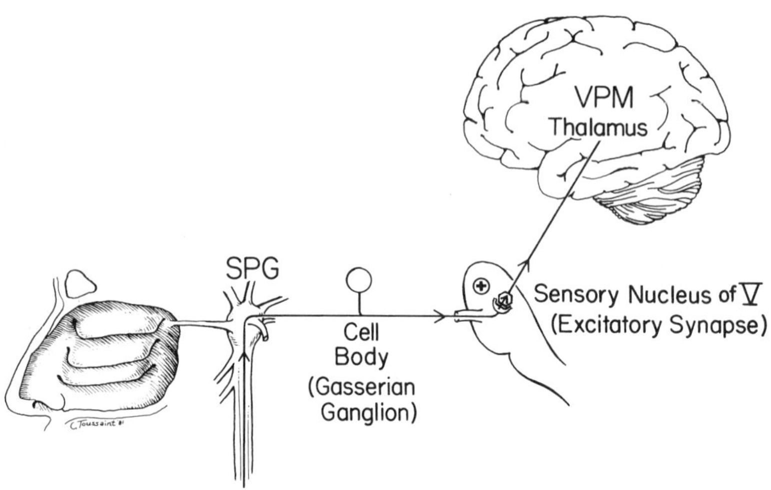

Figure 9-3A Sensory root of the sphenopalatine ganglion, through the trigeminal nerve, projecting to venteroposteromedial thalamic nucleus (VPM).

The parasympathetic root is essentially limited to the superficial petrosal nerve, the connection between the sphenopalatine ganglion and the facial nerve. Here, there are axons arising from cell bodies in the medulla oblongata which synapse on postganglionic cells in the sphenopalatine ganglion whose fibers are distributed widely over the nasal cavity, nasopharynx, palate, and orbit (see Figure 9-3B). Branches to the lacrimal gland account for the profuse lacrimation which may be seen immediately following physical stimulation of the sphenopalatine ganglion.

The sympathetic root of the sphenopalatine ganglion is the great deep petrosal nerve which is essentially an extension of the cervical sympathetic chain via the carotid plexus. Cell bodies in the ventral horn of the thoracolumbar spinal cord send fibers, either directly or via cervical ganglion synapse, some of which course through the sphenopalatine ganglion on their way to the periphery, and others which synapse in the

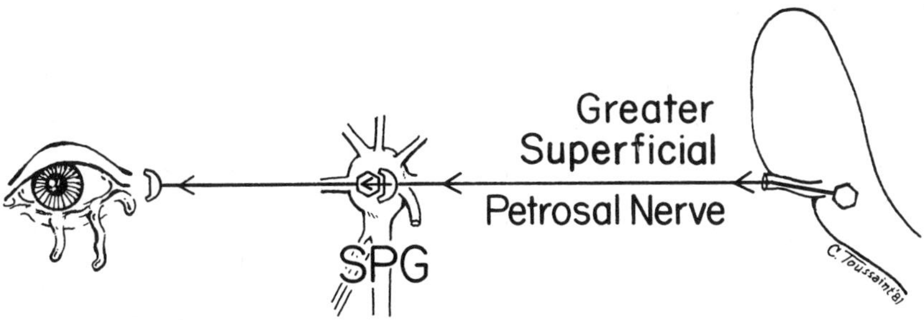

Figure 9-3B Parasympathetic root of sphenopalatine ganglion (SPG) from facial nerve via greater superficial petrosal nerve, with synapse at SPG, on to periphery (ie, lacrimal gland, as shown here).

sphenopalatine ganglion. There are also sensory afferent cells with cell bodies in dorsal roots of the spinal cord which synapse on interneurons and ventral horn sympathetic cells reflexly, whose peripheral axons course through the sphenopalatine ganglion (see Figure 9-3C). Anatomically, this interposes the sphenopalatine ganglion in a sympathetic reflex arc which loops between the thoracolumbar spinal cord and the head.

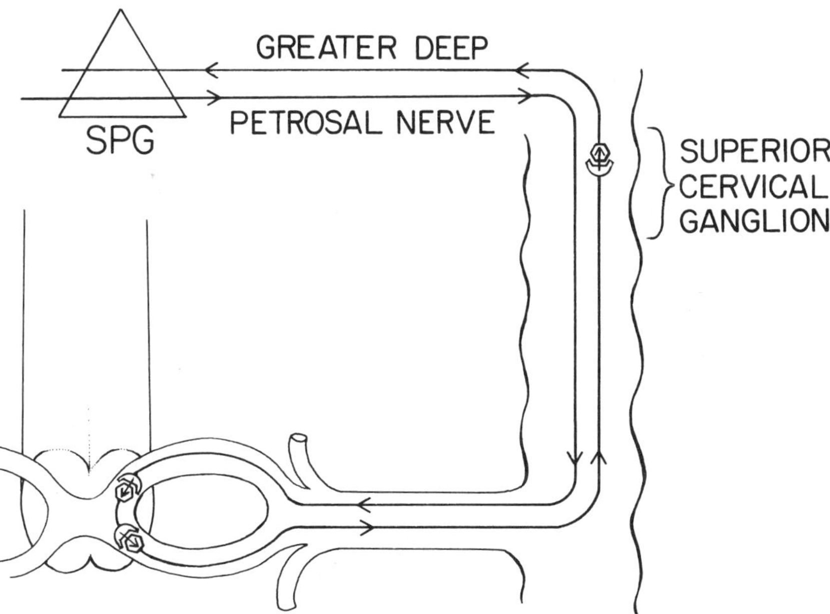

Figure 9-3C Sympathetic root of sphenopalatine ganglion (SPG), showing involvement in sympathetic reflex arc at level of spinal cord (lower left).

Zacharias (cited in Rosen et al, 1940) at Columbia University has described direct branches from the sphenopalatine ganglion to the anterior pituitary gland in his paper on pseudopregnancy following extirpation of the sphenopalatine ganglion in the rat, implying that the sphenopalatine ganglion has a tonic inhibitory influence on secretion of pituitary hormones which are now felt to include endorphins, the proposed endogenous peptide opiate agonists.

Technique

Sphenopalatine ganglion block consists of a simple topical anesthetization of the sphenopalatine ganglion through the nasal route as follows. The tips of four fine flexible Turnbull nasal applicators are covered with small bits of cotton and dipped into an anesthetic solution. A cotton tipped applicator is passed along the upper border of the inferior turbinate bone and directed backward and downward until the upper posterior wall of the pharynx is reached. Another applicator is directed along the upper border of the middle turbinate until the tip comes in contact with the sphenoid bone about a quarter of an inch external to the nasal septum. The same procedure is carried out on the opposite side (see Figure 9-4). The applicators are left in place for 30 min.

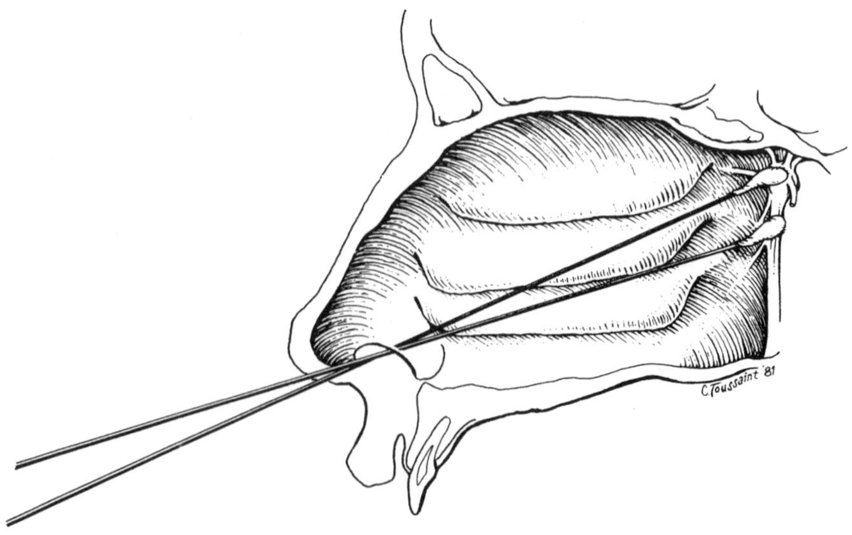

Figure 9-4 Technique of passage of cotton-tipped applicators to sphenopalatine ganglion using turbimate bones as guidelines.

From this position the anesthetic can diffuse approximately 5 mm and block the ganglion noninvasively and safely without any puncture or injection. Common side effects are a sensation of numbness in the back of the throat, a bitter taste in the mouth (secondary to dripping of the medication from the nasopharynx), and brief lacrimation. Patients occasionally report mild lightheadedness which always resolves within 30 min of termination of treatment. The best anesthetic for this procedure has proven to be cocaine because of its profound local anesthesia and rapid onset of action in the concentrations used. The total amount of cocaine on the applicators (0.2 to 0.4 cc of a 10% solution) is insufficient to produce central nervous system stimulation, and drug dependence has not been observed. Other topical local anesthetics are equally effective, but take much longer to have an analgesic effect. The only contraindication to this procedure is known hypersensitivity to the anesthetic used.

History

The history of sphenopalatine ganglion block dates to 1909 when Greenfield Sluder, clinical professor and director of the department of otolaryngology at Washington University School of Medicine, first described in a monograph the syndrome which bears his name, also known as "lower half headache" or "sphenopalatine neuralgia." This syndrome is characterized by unilateral pain at the root of the nose extending to the maxilla, mastoid, and occiput with radiation to the neck, shoulder, and in some cases as far down as the fingertips. Pain is often accompanied by salivation, lacrimation, and rhinorrhea. This syndrome probably has considerable overlap with pain syndromes now felt to be vasospastic in etiology, including cluster headache and migraine variants. Sluder emphasized that all of these symptoms and signs were remedied by blocking the sphenopalatine ganglion by application of cocaine solution or other topical anesthetic. In severe cases, he used 2% silver nitrate solution for more lasting effect, but cautioned against undesirable side effects of this method including mucosal atrophy.

In 1925 Simon Ruskin, who was best known for his invention of such pharmaceuticals as calcium ascorbate and procaine penicillin, turned his attention to this procedure and was the first to fully recognize its far reaching applications. He recommended the topical anesthetization of the sphenopalatine ganglion through the nasal route for control of painful vascular and muscle spasm, which he believed accounted for his observation that this treatment relieved a wide variety of symptoms including facial neuralgia, myalgic nodules (trigger points) in the trapezius and sternocleidomastoid muscles, headache, dysmenorrhea, and lumbago (lumbosacral strain). He noted that "it is almost unbelievable that the pain of sciatica which has resisted every form of therapy should yield within a few minutes to local application of cocaine in the nose."

Ruskin was not alone in utilizing this technique for treatment of muscle spasms at a distance. In 1931, Byrd reported treating low back strain, sciatica, asthma and angina. Heitger reported its use in brachial neuritis in 1925. In 1930, Byrd and Byrd reported a lengthy list of conditions with over 10,000 treatments having been given in 2000 patients. They indicated that lumbago was relieved in three-fourths of the cases. The last extensive case reports appeared in 1948 when Amster presented 103 case reports, using sphenopalatine ganglion block with pontocaine or cocaine, the bulk of which were made up of patients with lumbosacral or sacroiliac pain. He noted relief of pain and spasm in approximately 90% of his cases. Since that time one of the authors (MR) an otolaryngologist, has had the most extensive experience with this technique and has used it to treat patients with a wide variety of painful conditions. The greatest success has been noted with acute and chronic low back pain of multiple etiologies (muscular, discogenic, arthritic, and metastatic), sciatica, spastic torticollis, and refractory cluster headache. Before the technique became widely known in New York City, the patient population undergoing sphenopalatine ganglion block tended to be made up of those having symptoms refractory to conventional treatment, usually referred by neurologists or orthopedists as a last resort prior to surgery or referred following surgical failure or relapse. Great individual variation in patients' response time and degree of response has been seen; yet, the typical patient with chronic pain receiving an initial course of daily sphenopalatine ganglion block has some relief after the first few treatments and then progressively more complete and long-lasting relief until symptoms are minimal or absent without further therapy. In some patients there was nearly complete or complete relief after only one treatment, a state which can be maintained after completion of a one- to two-week course of follow-up treatments.

As more people in the professional community became aware of these successes, a shift was seen in the patient population with referrals being made earlier in a patient's course and with a growing number of patients, either themselves physicians or lay people having heard about the technique from others with similar problems, who presented with acute lumbosacral strain either untreated or simply dissatisfied with results of bedrest, analgesics, and muscle relaxants. Compared to the patients with chronic pain, these patients have a higher success rate and in many cases a dramatic response with complete lasting relief of pain and muscle spasm on the first treatment, with return to full function without further therapy. Patients are encouraged to continue their daily activities, with the exception of activities which aggravate the symptoms, and it is of interest that without any adjunctive measures (bedrest, cervical collar, back brace) it is highly unusual for a patient's condition to worsen on therapy.

Current Investigations

On the basis of these successes, a prospective double-blind clinical trial of sphenopalatine ganglion blockade in acute low back pain was initiated in 1981 through the Boston University School of Medicine and Department of Medicine at Boston City Hospital and is still in progress. Patients 18 to 65 years of age with low back pain for one week or less and pain free for at least one month prior to the acute episode are recruited from the emergency room, orthopedic clinic, and medical clinic, and after giving informed consent, undergo a thorough medical evaluation to exclude nonmusculoskeletal etiologies of back pain. Patients must have objective signs of musculoskeletal derangement and/or neurologic impairment. Patients then complete a visual analog questionnaire giving a semiquantitative subjective estimate of degree of pain and functional impairment and undergo a standardized battery of physical tests for muscle spasm, sciatic irritation, range of spinal motion, and ease of ambulation. Following this, they undergo either sphenopalatine ganglion block with 10% cocaine solution or a sham procedure with water as placebo. After 30 min, the questionnaire and tests are repeated. Preliminary results in the pilot group of 15 patients were encouraging, showing a strong trend toward treatment effect vs placebo. In the treatment group, 27% of patients were unchanged and 73% were improved, including 45% with marked to complete improvement after a single application. In the control group, 25% were improved and 75% were unchanged. In terms of analog scale grading in response to specific questions the differences were even larger. For example, in the question that compared severity of pain before and after treatment, the active treatment group showed an average of 51% improvement compared to 8% for the placebo group. When asked to estimate overall improvement on a 100-mm analog scale, the treatment group averaged 50 mm compared to 12 mm for the placebo group, with similar scores for separate estimates of improvement in pain alone and in mobility alone. The numbers are too small to draw statistical conclusions from the pilot study, but the trends are encouraging and work is in progress to study a large group of 100 patients, using the same methods.

Yang et al, at the College of Physicians and Surgeons, Columbia University, have recently reported statistically significant reduction in experimental pain (ischemic tourniquet pain in healthy volunteers) following application of 30 mg of cocaine to the area of the sphenopalatine ganglion compared to saline placebo controls in a 16-patient double-blind trial. These effects were without any measurable change in patients' affect or level of consciousness.

Dr. Edwin Goodman in the Department of Surgery at Columbia Presbyterian Hospital has reported personal experience with 200 patients with chronic pain of multiple etiologies, estimating a 90% response rate. Reder and Goodman have had a growing experience with patients suffering from pain of visceral involvement or bony metastasis from malignant tumor, including pancreatic carcinoma, bronchogenic carcinoma, prostatic carcinoma, and multiple myeloma, and have found that sphenopalatine ganglion block given on daily or every other day basis greatly reduces the requirement for narcotics and other analgesics, allowing improvement in mobility free from pain and overall quality of life without the undesirable CNS depressant effects of opiates.

The analgesic and antispasmodic effects of sphenopalatine ganglion block appear to be somewhat nonspecific, with new applications still being discovered. In addition to the more familiar indications, low back pain, sciatica, spastic torticollis, cluster headache, tic douloureux, Sluder's syndrome, and causalgia, there are an increasing number of anecdotal successes reported with other conditions characterized by smooth or skeletal muscle spasm, including refractory Raynaud's phenomenon, dysmenorrhea, temperomandibular joint dysfunction, chronic hiccup, bronchospasm, and painful spasm in multiple sclerosis.

Discussion

A mechanism to explain these empiric observations has not been conclusively demonstrated. As alluded to earlier, there are multiple candidates for an anatomic substrate for these observed phenomena.

The connections of the sphenopalatine ganglion to the hypothalamic-pituitary axis are of interest in terms of a potential neurohumoral hypothesis, which should be easily tested as assays for endorphin activity are improved.

A second possible mechanism is suggested by the trigeminal connection, as described above, which may at least in the case of trigeminal and other cephalic neuralgias allow the sphenopalatine ganglion to alter the state of a pain gate-control system operating at the level of the sensory nucleus of the trigeminal nerve.

Third, the connections between the sphenopalatine ganglion and afferent neurons which run in the sympathetic chain with their cell bodies in the dorsal root and appearing to be involved in a reflex sympathetic arc are also of interest in this regard. It is not difficult to imagine that such neurons could synapse on interneurons involved in pain perception and the maintenance of muscle spasm secondary to it. At the International Symposium on Pain in 1974, several papers were presented concerning pain and the autonomic nervous system. Gross quoted

Bonica's observation that it is "lack of neurotomal distribution that has delayed recognition of this group of disorders as clinical entities." He went on to quote Leriche, who observed that certain types of pain disappeared after localized resection of the sympathetic chain and that stimulation of the cervical sympathetic trunk during surgery produced "very strong painful anxiety and produced strong pains in the lower jaw teeth and behind the ear on the same side." These radiations did not correspond to the known topography of spinal nerves. Citing these and many other studies, Gross concluded that the sympathetic pain syndromes corresponded to vascular zone topography. Melzack, originator of the gate-control theory of pain perception, commented in 1972 that "the sympathetic nervous system contributes in some way to all of these pain states," but implied that specific knowledge in this area is sorely lacking.

Procacci and co-workers reported a study of cutaneous pain threshold changes after sympathetic block in reflex dystrophies. He indicated that in the opinion of some investigators an abnormal sympathetic reflex activity is present in many diseases differently classified. This activity induces and maintains trophic disturbances, pain, and other sensory alterations. This mechanism is operant, for instance, in some limb vascular diseases and in some rheumatic diseases, as in muscular rheumatism with myalgic spots (fibrositis), often having the well-known characteristics of trigger points. They carried out pharmacologic block of the sympathetic chain ipsilateral to the affected limb and found that not only was the causalgic pain relieved but the trigger points became less painful to pressure or completely disappeared, even in the limb contralateral to the sympathetic block. They pointed out that recent concepts regarding sympathetic control are that:

1. Efferent sympathetic discharge is under the control of ipsilateral and contralateral neuronal systems located at different levels in the CNS. Every change of the afferent cutaneous, muscular, or visceral input to the CNS sets up variations of the sympathetic discharge through spinal, bulbar, and suprabulbar somato- and viscerosympathetic reflexes.
2. The efferent sympathetic fibers to somatic and visceral structures and most of the visceral afferents pass through the sympathetic ganglia, as well as some afferent somatic fibers.

They concluded that pharmacological block of the sympathetic ganglia produces an interruption of the efferent sympathetic and afferent visceral fibers of the blocked side. Their research also showed that the sympathetic system controls the cutaneous pain threshold and that sympathetic block induced changes not only in the skin but also in ipsi- and contralateral deep tissues "as shown by the disappearance or attenuation of the muscular trigger points." At this time our discussion of these potential mechanisms is purely speculative and careful physiologic testing will be required to elucidate the true basis of the observed effects.

An argument that the effect of sphenopalatine ganglion block is due to psychological factors has been raised. This is unlikely in that in many cases the most elaborate types of treatment given to patients on numerous instances and over prolonged periods of time did not effect the remissions that occurred dramatically with sympathetic blocking. It is certainly true that many of the symptoms amenable to this treatment can on occasion be due to psychosomatic dysfunction. The important point here is that almost all if not all psychosomatic symptoms are probably mediated by the autonomic nervous system, and if in the cases cited by many authors the symptoms were of psychogenic etiology, the treatment by sympathetic block probably works by disrupting the physiological substrata rather than by suggestion.

In conclusion, sphenopalatine ganglion block is a safe, noninvasive procedure easily, painlessly, and rapidly performed in the outpatient setting which is potentially of benefit to any patient with pain, in particular, that due to muscle spasm, vasospasm, neuralgia, or reflex sympathetic dystrophy. The technique does not require the hand of an otolaryngologist, but should be learned from a practitioner who has had direct experience with it. Patients should be started on a course of daily applications. Treatment course must be tailored to individual patients, but certain general guidelines apply. In patients for whom relief initially lasts less than six hours, treatments can be increased to twice daily over the first few days. In acute conditions, one week of treatments is a reasonable therapeutic trial, with little hope of later success if absolutely no improvement has occurred by that time. In chronic conditions, two to three weeks of treatment should be given in all cases, and if any improvement is noted during this period, treatments should be continued as there is an excellent chance of remission.

Further clinical research will be required to establish sphenopalatine ganglion block as a first-line treatment for many of the conditions listed above, and considering its relative safety and lack of significant side effects, this would represent an attractive alternative in most cases.

In patients with pain refractory to conventional modalities, a trial of sphenopalatine ganglion block is certainly indicated, as it is impossible to predict which patients will respond and the risk is practically nonexistent, based on vast prior experience.

BIBLIOGRAPHY

Amster JL: Sphenopalatine block for relief of lumbosacral pain. *NY State J Med* 1948;48:2475–2480.

Bonica J: Autonomic innervation and nerve block. *Anesthesiology* 1968;29: 793-813.
Byrd H: Sphenopalatine test. *J Mich Med Soc* 1930;29:294–298.
Byrd H, Byrd W: Sphenopalatine phenomena; present status of knowledge. *Arch Inter Med* 1930;46:1026–1038.
Gross D: International Symposium on Pain, Seattle, Washington. *Adv Neurol* 1974;4:93.
Leriche R, quoted by Gross D: La chirurgie de la douleur—*Adv Neurol* 1974; 4:93.
Melzack R: Mechanisms of pathologic pain, in Critchley M, O'Leary, Jennett (eds): *Scientific Foundations of Neurology.* London, Heinemann, 1974.
Procaci P, Francini F, Zoppi M, et al: Cutaneous pain threshold changes after sympathetic block in reflex dystrophies. *Pain* 1975;1:167–175.
Rosen S, et al: Naso-genital relationship in the rat. *Endrocrinology* 1940;27: 463–468.
Ruskin AP: Sphenopalatine ganglion: Its role in pain spasm and the rage reaction and possible relationship to acupuncture. *Acupunc Electrother Res Int J* 1979;4:91–103.
Ruskin SL: Contributions to the study of the sphenopalatine ganglion. *Laryngoscope* 1925;25:87–108.
Ruskin SL: Technic of sphenopalatine ganglion therapy. *Eye Ear Nose Throat Monthly* 1951;30:28–31.
Sluder G: The anatomical and clinical relations of the sphenopalatine ganglion to the nose. *NY State J Med* 1909;90:293–298.
Sluder G: The syndrome of sphenopalatine ganglion neuralgia. *Am J Med Sci* 1910;111:868–878.
Sluder G: *Nasal Neurology, Headaches and Eye Disorders.* St. Louis, CV Mosby, 1927.
Yang JC, Clark WC, Dooley JC, et al: Effect of intranasal cocaine on experimental pain in man. *Anesth Anal* 1982;61:358–361.

SELECTED READINGS

Byrd H: Nasal ganglion or switchboard test; working device. *Med J Rec* 1928; 128:68–71.
Dock G: Sluder's nasal ganglion syndrome and its relation to internal medicine. *JAMA* 1929;93:750–753.
Gundrum LK: Migraine controlled through nasal ganglion. *Arch Otolaryngol* 1928;8:564–566.
Haugen: Autonomic nervous system. *Anesthesiology* 1968;29:785–792.
Janzen: *Pain*. Stuttgart, Thieme, 1972.
Kunkel RS: A complexity of headaches. *Emer Med* 1981;13:24.
Luedde WH: Relation of Meckel's ganglion to tension. *IMJ* 1941;79:199–209.
Ruskin SL: Contributions to the study of the sphenopalatine ganglion. *Laryngoscope* 1925;3–24.
Ruskin SL: The control of muscle spasm and arthritic pain through sympathetic block at the nasal ganglion and the use of the adenylic nucleotide. *Am J Dig Dis* 1946;13:311–320.
Stewart D, Lambert V: Sphenopalatine ganglion. *J Laryngol Otol* 1930;45: 753–771.
Stewart D, Lambert V: Further observations on sphenopalatine ganglion. *J Laryngol Otol* 1934;49:19–22.
White JC: *Pain, Control and Mechanisms.* Springfield, Charles C. Thomas, 1955.

10 Nerve Blocks

John Rybock

Interrupting a nerve's function by injecting a local anesthetic or a neurodestructive agent can provide important diagnostic information or therapeutic relief in some patients with chronic pain. However, nerve blocks used without careful regard to selection of patients, technique and follow-up evaluation are likely to confuse the clinical picture and interfere with an adequate resolution of the patient's problem. Each factor must be carefully evaluated before nerve blockade can have a justifiable role in pain therapy.

Selection of Patients

It must be recognized that nerve blocks are of minimal efficacy for the majority of patients with chronic pain. Sequentially blocking each nerve that in part serves an area of pain neither improves the understanding of a patient's pain nor leads to a useful therapy. Only after adequately evaluating the patient's pain problem both organically and psychologically can a decision be made regarding the potential usefulness of nerve blocks; a reasonable working diagnosis must be developed. In only a few such diagnoses can nerve blocks aid in confirming the diagnosis or in providing therapy.

Perhaps the greatest limitation in using nerve blocks in pain diagnosis is that the results can only be evaluated through the patient's report. The physician must know enough about the patient and his means of describing his pain, as well as how the pain varies over time and with various activities, to be able to interpret the patient's report.

As has been stressed in other sections of this book, the patient describing chronic pain is not providing an objective assessment of a nociceptive input, but is expressing chronic suffering in a way which is psychologically acceptable. The relative contributions of organic dysfunction, psychological abnormalities, and social factors in the unitary complaint of "pain" are seldom obvious upon early contact with the patient. Assuming an important direct relationship between nociceptive input and reported pain leads to the premature use of nerve blocks, which may be harmful. A successful block, notably reducing the underlying nociceptive input, may not yield a positive report by the patient if marked nonorganic factors are present. Conversely, some patients may report good results even with inadequate blocks for a variety of reasons. In either case, the physician receives incorrect information which may either prevent the application of the appropriate interventional methods when the proper stage in therapy arrives, or lead to inappropriate therapy which only aggravates the patient's problem. The early application of nerve blocks allows both the physician and patient to focus on organic factors alone and delay recognition of potentially more important psychological and social factors. Once the psychological and social aspects of the patient's problems have been adequately identified and appropriately dealt with, the organic aspect of the patient's problem becomes critical in making a decision to undertake nerve-block therapy.

A tentative diagnosis or a limited differential diagnosis must be made on the basis of clinical evidence. If such a diagnosis includes injury to a single nerve or root, posttraumatic sympathetic dystrophy, myofascial syndrome, or facet syndrome, then a potential for nerve blocking exists. Except in rare instances, other diagnoses do not call for nerve blockade, either for diagnosis or treatment.

In many cases of single nerve injury, the diagnosis is made by means other than nerve block. For example, carpal tunnel syndrome or tardy ulnar palsy are best confirmed by nerve conduction studies. In nerves not easily studied by this technique, such as the lateral femoral cutaneous nerve causing meralgia paresthetica, a block can be diagnostic. Also, in cases of persistent sciatica following lumbar discectomy, selective blockade can confirm single root involvement and lead to appropriate surgical exploration or dorsal rhizotomy. In some cases, blockade can be of therapeutic value when a despository steroid or neurolytic agent is added.

Posttraumatic sympathetic dystrophy is characterized by a diffuse burning dysesthesia which usually does not follow a single nerve or dermatomal pattern. It often occurs insidiously following an often minor distal extremity injury, although in its most classic form follows a major nerve injury; sympathetic hyperactivity in the extremity is the common component. The affected area is characteristically cool and secondary trophic changes in the skin, hair, and nails occur, as well as osteoporosis. Although an accurate clinical diagnosis can usually be made, relief following sympathetic blockade is confirmatory. In addition, for reasons poorly understood, repeated sympathetic blockade with local anesthetic can sometimes lead to long-lasting relief.

Facet joint dysfunction apparently causes some cases of nondiscogenic back pain. Traumatic arthritis of the facet joints, the only true diarthrodial joints in the spine, is thought to cause reflex muscle spasm, as well as pain referral into the hip or gluteal areas. The patient's pain can be reproduced by hyperextension of the lumbar spine, which compresses the facets. The diagnosis is made by pain relief following facet block, the injection of local anesthetic in a position which blocks the sensory fibers from the facet joint and capsule. If excellent pain relief occurs, facet denervation by thermal coagulation of the joint's nerve supply can be carried out. This is a specialized technique, requiring fluoroscopy and a radiofrequency electrode system; the technical aspects have been well defined by Long and Bogduk.

Myofascial syndrome is the least understood entity amenable to nerve blockade. This syndrome can affect any muscular area, although the shoulder girdle and paraspinal muscles are the most common sites of involvement. The basic complaint is dull aching pain not following a dermatomal or neural pattern, but often radiating into an extremity or into the head with subjective experiences of weakness and tingling, also not in a dermatomal pattern. The characteristic finding is the trigger point, a tender area within the substance of a muscle which is unusually firm to palpation, and which, when stimulated, often reproduces symptoms including the radiating sensations. It appears that trigger points are areas of overcontraction within a muscle which produce focal ischemia, increased pain, and further reflex contraction. Inflammatory changes, waxy degeneration of muscle fibers, and fibrosis have been demonstrated in such nodules. The radiating symptoms may represent referral along the myotome rather than the dermatome. Various forms of therapy, such as surface cooling or application of counterirritants, diathermy, and biofeedback have been utilized as therapy; it appears that the most prompt relief follows injection of local anesthetic agents into the trigger points, followed by stretching of the muscle by massage or active exercise. In theory, the pain provoking reflex contraction is blocked, and the muscle fibers may, in fact, be locally paralyzed, so that the fibrils may be restored to physiologic length and the flow of blood can again occur.

Often, repeated injections and stretching spaced over days to weeks are required to relieve the pain, particularly if the problem has been long standing and fibrosis has occurred.

Technique

To perform a useful block, the injection should be accurate, requiring a small amount of agent. Roughly aiming at a nerve and flooding the area with anesthetic yields an unpredictable blockade and often results in spread to adjacent nerves. This makes the results uninterpretable. For example, a well performed stellate block requires only 1 ml of agent, while a lumbar sympathetic block can be accomplished with 10 ml. Specific injection techniques will not be discussed here. Several textbooks on technique are available; Moore's textbook appears to be the most comprehensive and is currently our standard reference. It should be noted, however, that Moore's techniques do not use radiologic control. This is reasonable for many simple blocks which can be used at bedside, such as myofascial trigger point injections, stellate blocks, intercostal blocks, and blockade of the lateral femoral cutaneous nerve, but other blocks such as spinal root blocks and lumbar sympathetic blocks are so much more easily done with fluoroscopic control that the traditional techniques, using trigonometric methods, are unnecessary.

The blocking agent used depends upon the goals of the block. For most blocks, intermediate local anesthetic such as 1% lidocaine is preferred. This agent works promptly and is effective for several hours, which is adequate for most blocks. Occasionally, longer lasting blocks are desired in which case 0.5% bupivacaine can be used. Further prolongation of effect can be obtained by adding epinephrine to the blocking agent.

If temporary blocks with local anesthetics are beneficial, additional agents may be used to achieve a longer lasting effect. Phenol or alcohol have been traditionally used to cause neurocoagulation. Although still used occasionally for trigeminal branch or intercostal nerve blocks, nonselective neural destruction and adjacent tissue destruction make these agents less than ideal choices. We currently prefer differential thermocoagulation with a radiofrequency electrode if long lasting blockade is desired.

In cases where neural inflammation is suspected, such as persistent postsurgical lumbar radiculitis or lateral cutaneous nerve entrapment, injection of a depository steriod can provide long-lasting relief. Whether the benefit is derived from the steriod's anti-inflammatory action or from its mild neurotoxic properties is unclear.

Evaluation

No block can provide useful information if the practitioner is unable to carefully evaluate the result. There are two aspects in the evaluation of a nerve block, specifically confirmation of effectiveness of blockade of the desired nerve and it alone, and the effect of that blockade on the patient's pain complaint. Objective means must be used to confirm the effectiveness of the block at the neural level, for with even the best technique, adequate blockade may not be obtained. With sympathetic nerve blocks, assessment of temperature changes by touch or thermography as well as observation of visual signs of increased cutaneous circulation, can be used. With somatic nerve blocks, appropriate motor or sensory loss must be documented.

If an effective block can be confirmed, the patient's report must be carefully interpreted. Simply enquiring as to whether the block relieved the pain is insufficient. Many patients, even when apparently properly instructed, will report that the block was not helpful if the pain has returned at the time of questioning. Therefore, it is recommended that the patient be requested to record in writing at 15- to 30-minute intervals the level of his pain, the activities being performed at the time of observation, as well as any subjective changes such as weakness or numbness. These data, coupled with the knowledge of the patient's usual pain pattern, permit a reasonable assessment of the block.

Careful analysis requires the realization that many patients will slant reports of effectiveness in an attempt to please the physician. In addition, the placebo effect on pain can occur with nerve blocks as it does with other medications. If any doubt exists as to the true effectiveness of the block, the physician should be prepared to repeat the block several times, in some cases using blocking agents of different durations or using blockade of different nerves in subsequent blocks; in occasional complex cases, one might consider the use of a placebo injection.

Conclusions

For a limited group of patients with chronic pain, nerve blockade is extremely useful in diagnosis and treatment. However, one must avoid the tendency to use the nerve block early in the course of diagnosis in an attempt to "get to the bottom of the problem" quickly. Only after careful consideration of selection, technique, and evaluation can nerve blockade be utilized in the care of the individual patient.

BIBLIOGRAPHY

Cailliet R: *Soft Tissue Pain and Disability*. Philadelphia, FA Davis Co, 1977.

Long DM, Bogduk N: Percutaneous lumbar medial branch neurotomy. *Spine* 1980;5:193–200.

Moore D: *Regional Block,* ed 4. Springfield, Ill, Charles C Thomas, 1965.

Sola A: Myofascial trigger point therapy. *Res Staff Phys* 1981;27:38–45.

White J, Sweet W: *Pain and the Neurosurgeon*. Springfield, Ill, Charles C Thomas, 1969.

SECTION IV
Headaches

11 Mechanical (Structural) Headache

David A. Zohn

Within the framework of musculoskeletal pain disorders, headache might be approached in the context of these problems. Often the complaint of headache is simply a part of the larger picture of musculoskeletal pain as presented by many patients. This type of headache has been variously labeled tension headache, psychogenic headache, or muscle contraction headache. Although the latter term is better than either of the former, all are a misnomer. Indeed, there is a great deal of tension in these patients and a great deal of pathology in the muscles; however, the entire spine and all of its supporting structures can be a source of pathology leading to the complaint of headache. For that reason, the term "mechanical headache" appears more appropriate. Perhaps an even better term might be structural headache, since all of the spine and its supporting structures can produce pathology which will eventually lead to headache.

In the various texts on headache, it is generally agreed that up to 90% of the patients present with this type of problem. In the office of the family practitioner or internist, as opposed to the office of a neurologist or a neurosurgeon or in a headache clinic, it is probably an even higher percentage. Yet, in these texts the least information and the least amount of attention is paid to this type of headache. The discussion usually focuses on the psychological aspects and the necessity for psychotherapy. There is a brief discussion of drugs and a very superficial discussion of physical therapy (usually recommending the application of hot packs to the muscles), and some discussion of biofeedback. There is virtually no discussion of faulty mechanics or specific treatment of the pathology that does exist in the spine and its supporting structures. This is surprising since whatever the psychologic component to the problem, and it is large, the pain itself is arising from pathology in the tissues. This is real pathology, just as there is a real pathology in peptic ulcer disease and in ulcerative colitis, and all of the other illnesses which have a psychosomatic component. In diagnosing mechanical headache, one must take not only a good history but in the course of the physical examination one must also use the fingers instead of relying on x-ray films and laboratory studies; perhaps too many of us are not trained to use our hands to make a diagnosis in musculoskeletal problems. If it is accepted that there is organic pathology present, effective treatment can be begun with a combination of drugs, injections, and physical therapeutic means and psychotherapy when indicated.

For reasons which are unclear, mechanical headache problem appears predominantly in females. This is also true of myofascial pain, fibrositis, and muscular problems associated with the temporomandibular joint (TMJ) syndrome all of which, including mechanical headache, are poorly understood, offer no clear-cut laboratory clues, and are often refractory to treatment.

Anatomy and Mechanics

To further understand this type of headache it is necessary to present some background information on anatomy and mechanics. Upon examining the spine it is seen to be one unit, not the cervical, the thoracic, and the lumbar spine as we study it in medical school and the way we talk about it for convenience. It is one unit, and motion in one area produces motion in another area, however slight. Similarly, muscle contraction in one area produces muscle contraction in another area, and muscle pathology in one area may well lead to muscle pathology elsewhere. Therefore, one must look at the entire spine when looking at this problem.

From a mechanical standpoint, the spine is a flexible column of 24 blocks joined by muscles and ligaments, its role being to keep the trunk upright, resisting the effects of gravity. It also keeps the trunk in the midline, because this position produces the least amount of energy expenditure. On top of the spine is balanced a 10- to 12-pound ball, the skull. The spine also attempts to keep this ball in the midline for optimum binocular vision and minimal stimulation of the labyrinth, since chronic stimulation of the labyrinth and chronic production of righting reflexes causes chronic contraction of the muscles.

It is helpful, when looking at the skull balanced on top of the spine, to think of it as a lever system. The fulcrum is at the atlanto-occipital joints. The center of gravity is at the sella turcica which is anterior to the atlanto-occipital joints, and thus the weight of the skull forces the head forward. This is readily apparent when someone in the sitting position starts to nod, with the result that the head falls forward instead of backwards. The counterbalancing forces for the weight of the skull are the posterior cervical muscles. Anything which forces the head forward more than usual requires increased countervailing forces by the posterior cervical muscles. Many positions have as their common denominators the fact that the head is thrust forward for a prolonged period of time, eg, sitting propped up on pillows while reading or watching television, awkward work positions, sloping shoulders and increased lumbar lordosis which causes a compensatory increased cervical lordosis. All of these cause the head to be thrust forward and thus the posterior cervical muscles must work harder in order to keep the head erect. It is the chronic contraction of these muscles which causes trouble.

Although anatomically we think of the spine as being made up of a number of vertebrae, from the functional standpoint it is composed of what are called functional units. These units consist of the disc, the vertebrae, and the supporting ligaments and muscles. The different portions of the vertebrae have different mechanical functions. The body of the vertebrae (as well as the intervening disc) is the weight-bearing portion. The type of stress placed on this portion is twofold: compression stress and shearing stress. Some shearing stress is also borne by the pars interarticularis while the posterior elements (the facet joints) have as their function the guiding of movements between adjacent vertebrae. This is all true in the intact functional unit, but changes in one portion of the unit can lead to altered function in other portions of the unit. The ligaments consist of the anterior longitudinal ligament, the ligamentum flavum, the interspinous ligaments, and the supraspinous ligaments. This last ligament is known in the neck as the ligamentum nuchae. The anterior and posterior longitudinal ligaments are pain sensitive, whereas the others are not. There are also facet joints and the joint capsules which are likewise pain sensitive, as is the dura mater around the nerve roots.

Surrounding these structures are the muscles, the description of which is usually approached in two quite different ways: very complicated or very simple. The complicated way is to divide and then further divide the myriad layers and groups of muscles to the point of total confusion. The simple way, and in all likelihood the way for most physicians, is to simply ignore them. A path midway between the two can be taken with benefit. These can be regarded as four separate layers of muscles (only three layers in the lumbar spine) with the deepest layer the shortest and, as the layers become superficial, extending over longer and longer segments. At the deepest level the muscles extend from one to four segments and are variously called the multifidi, rotatories, and interspinales. In the cervical spine, our area of particular concern, they have different names and they are named according to the direction in which their fibers run, the rectus (which means straight) major and minor, and obliquus (which run in the obvious fashion) superior and inferior. These all attach along the nuchal line. The importance of these muscles is that they are the fine tuning muscles of the head which, by contraction, insure that the head is evenly balanced and carried in the fashion previously described.

The next more superficial layer is the semispinalis muscle which extends over four to six segments. The muscle that we are most concerned about in this layer in the neck is the semispinalis capitis muscle and capitis, of course, means that it attaches to the skull. This muscle is pierced by the great occipital nerve and this has clinical importance. Overlying this layer is the erector spinae muscle group which traverses many segments. It is divided into three longitudinal groups, the most lateral being the iliocostalis, then the longissimus and most medially, the spinalis. The one group of muscles in this layer in the neck which we are most concerned about is the splenius capitis. The splenius capitis muscle arises from the lower half of the ligamentum of nuchae, the spinous process of C-7, and the upper three or four thoracic vertebrae and inserts laterally onto the mastoid process and occipital bone. In contrast to most of the muscles of the back, these fibers run obliquely. The importance of this muscle is in its being a very common site of trigger points and, therefore, a very common source of neck pain. It is important to palpate this muscle carefully during the examination of the neck in order to detect pathology. Overlying this layer of muscle is a fourth layer, not truly back muscles at all, but muscles of the upper trunk and shoulder girdle. These include the trapezius and the sternocleidomastoid muscle. The sternocleido-mastoid muscle is usually thought of as an anterior muscle, but the upper portion of this muscle becomes posterior as it inserts on the mastoid process and the occiput, and, therefore, becomes the most superficial portion of the posterior muscles.

The nerve supply of the functional unit is largely from the recurrent nerve of Luschka. In the neck, the nerves which have clinical significance in this context are the greater and lesser occipital nerves. The great occipital nerve is the medial branch of the dorsal ramus of C-2, while the lesser occipital nerve arises from the ventral ramus of C-2 and C-3. Both provide sensory innervation to the upper portion of the neck and to the posterior portion of the scalp. These nerves have interconnections with cranial nerve V, at least partially explaining some of the peculiar path distributions in patients with this type of headache. Most important of all, these nerves pierce the posterior neck muscles and, therefore, are subject to entrapment by muscle spasm.

The atlanto-occipital joint is an important joint which was alluded to earlier when it was mentioned that these joints are the fulcrum on which the skull balances. These are large rocker joints which are concerned primarily with the nodding movements of the head, but because they are large joints which are on a horizontal plane (universal joints) they participate in all other motions of the neck. Problems of loss of motion here, which can be called joint dysfunction, either primary or secondary, contribute to the problem of headache and must be looked for and eradicated in the treatment of this type of headache.

It is worth commenting about leg length discrepancy and its importance (surprisingly) in the production of headache. The spine normally arises at right angles from the horizontal sacrum and descends in the midline. If there is a leg length discrepancy, in order to keep the spine and the center of gravity in the midline a scoliosis develops. This curve starts at the lumbar spine with a compensatory curve in the thoracic spine. These curves must be kept in place by contraction of the muscles, with associated chronic stress on the ligaments supporting the spine. The muscles and ligaments of the neck are included in the stress, leading to pathologic changes in these tissues and subsequently to headache. It needs to be emphasized that these curves need not be, and indeed are usually not, the gross curves requiring orthopedic intervention. Therefore, it is appropriate in examining a patient with headache to check for this problem also.

A few general comments about anatomy and mechanics would be in order. It should be noted that normal muscles do not contract constantly: they contract and they relax. If there is a constant contraction of the muscle, pathologic changes develop in these muscles. There is an interesting phenomenon in the spine and that is that we as individuals are unable to isolate motion of a single moving segment of the spine. For instance, we are well aware if we put our hand behind our back that the joints of the fingers are bent, that the wrist is bent, or that the elbow is bent. But who has any concept that C-4 is rotated on C-5, or L-3 is flexed in relation to L-4? We do not appear to have any concept in the spine of where we are in space except over long segments of the spine. There seems to be a lack of proprioception, and this may be a source of many problems in back and neck pain, because the brain may be getting false information about the actual relation of the spinal segments. Therefore, minimal unguarded movements such as turning to put something in the wastebasket or bending to tie shoelaces results in an acute wry neck or an acute back spasm. If the brain is unaware that the spinal segments are already approximated and the attached muscles are already shortened, then a volley of impulses from the brain instructing the muscles to contract may produce tremendous spasm of these muscles which are already shortened.

It should be noted that the final common path of pathology in the musculoskeletal system is loss of motion. Therefore, in addition to whatever else is treated, restoration of motion is essential. This is carried out through the treatment program, supplemented at home by the patient and, in chronic problems, followed through by the patient after cessation of formal treatment.

Trigger Points and Myofascial Pain

This pathologic condition, often overlooked by physicians, is a common source of mechanical headache. A trigger point is an irritable focus in a muscle with a referred pattern of pain. This referred pattern of pain may be in the soft tissues around the trigger point or may be completely distant from it and not related to it in any contiguous fashion. Myofascial pain is the name commonly given to this entity. The pattern of referred pain does not follow any root or peripheral nerve distribution and because of this a label of a functional disorder may be wrongly applied to the patient. It should be noted that the majority of headaches caused by trigger points arise from outside the head, in the neck and upper back. The pathophysiology of the trigger point is in debate. Some researchers have reported pathologic changes and others have found nothing. It is widely believed that the irritable focus is an abnormally firing muscle spindle, but this awaits pathologic confirmation. Electromyographic findings in trigger points are likewise in debate; those people who have found electromyographic changes report them in only a small percentage of the cases which they see which makes one wonder how real this finding is.

The trigger point may be either primary or secondary. As an example of a secondary trigger point, one may have an unrelated problem such as a true herniated nucleus pulposus with true radiculitis and yet have trigger points in the root distribution. Understanding this explains why perfectly valid surgery is performed, the pathologic disc material is removed, and yet the pain persists. This pain may have absolutely nothing to do with the root compression by the disc material but may be due to a trigger point in the muscles which has not been eradicated. Therefore, it is important to understand that trigger points may arise de noveau or may be a secondary phenomenon which has to be treated in conjunction with other pathologic processes.

The etiology of the trigger point is usually said to be trauma, tension, infection, and chronic overuse; metabolic, endocrine, and nutritional causes have also been included, but it is not clear that it is valid to do so. It is important to note that there is segmental spasm of the muscle surrounding the trigger point. This means that the entire muscle is not in spasm, rather, just the segment of muscle surrounding the trigger point. One cannot observe this spasm; it can be detected only by palpation. This shortened segment is painful and prevents normal function of the entire muscle. And, because abnormal muscle is unable to perform the normal functions of relaxing and contracting, it accumulates metabolites. This, in turn, may set up satellite trigger points which in their turn cause further problems.

Trigger points are tender to pressure and they exhibit a positive jump sign. The jump sign is often described as observing the patient jump as the painful trigger point is palpated. What is really meant by that sign is that by placing the affected muscle on the stretch and by strumming across the segment in spasm, that portion of the muscle can be observed to twitch.

In view of the fact that there are thus far no good laboratory methods to identify trigger points (and myofascial pain), it is not surprising that several different methods are being evaluated. One is a pressure meter which records the amount of pressure that a patient can tolerate before exhibiting pain. This is applied over a suspected trigger point and the corresponding opposite side is also measured. If there is a significant numerical difference, then this is considered to be a valid trigger point. A second method is to observe the electrical properties of the trigger point by means of electrical stimulation. A third method, thermography, observes the pattern of heat output from the affected area. An area of increased heat output which does not follow dermatomal distribution may represent an active trigger point and its area of referred pain.

The treatment of trigger points will be discussed in a later section but at this time two principles of treatment of trigger points should be mentioned. First, one must block the pain from the trigger point and therefore break the cycle of pain. Second, one must stretch the segment of muscle surrounding the trigger point which is in spasm and restore the normal resting length of that segment of muscle in spasm. Often patients come from other physicians who say "Yes, you have trigger points, but there is no point in treating them because they always come back!" That is true. If one does not stretch out the associated segment of muscle in spasm, the trigger point will recur and one will have this as a chronic problem. These two factors go together, blocking the pain and thereby breaking the cycle of pain, and then restoring the normal resting length for that muscle.

Etiology

The first cause of this type of headache is trauma. Macro- and microtrauma should be differentiated. Macrotrauma is obvious, the most common cause being the soft tissue injuries associated with automobile accidents. Headache may result from entrapment of the great occipital nerve by spasm of the posterior cervical muscles through which it passes. However, this is a far less common mechanism than the establishment of trigger points in the musculature which refers pain to the head. On the other hand, microtrauma is the chronic recurring low-grade trauma in, for example, the patient with poorly fitting bifocals or in the patient with an occupation which causes the head to be constantly tilted such as the salesman who uses the telephone all day. The altered mechanics of the musculature set up trigger points in them which in turn refer pain to the head.

Degenerative joint disease causes headaches which result from altered mechanics. As the disc degenerates, its height decreases producing secondary changes in the functional unit, because the anterior portion of the functional unit which bears the stress of weight bearing is no longer able to adequately perform that function. This throws excessive stress on the posterior or guiding elements which are the facet joints. In turn, this makes the whole functional unit more susceptible to trauma, either major or minor. What results is the development of a low-grade synovitis in the facet joints and/or chronic ligamentous and muscle strain or both. This, in turn, produces pain and limitation of motion. The limitation of motion and the pain produces fixed shortening of the muscles, ligaments, and joint capsules. This loss of motion produces pathological alteration in these tissues because they are not able to perform the normal toilet of ridding themselves of catabolites, and it is these catabolites which produce persistent pain.

It is important in degenerative joint disease not to rely on roentgenograms to make the diagnosis because the x-ray films of virtually 100 percent of the people over the age of 50 show some element of degenerative joint disease. They all have some narrowing of the disc, some lipping, or spur formation, and many even have encroachment upon the neural foramina or some element of subluxation. Rather, there are important points in the history such as pain, loss of motion, crepitus, morning stiffness, increased symptomatology with alteration in the barometric pressure, and in the physical examination which include loss of range of motion, tenderness in the muscles, pain on stretching the muscles, and tenderness over the neural foramina, all of which are important clinical features in making the diagnosis.

Faulty posture and mechanics serve as both etiologic and perpetuating agents in this type of headache. Patients with large breasts, proper work habits, poorly fitting bifocals, and poor posture all have mechanical problems which need to be corrected. It is important to remember that depression alters posture. We somaticize how we feel, and the chronically depressed patient with the hunched back and sloped shoulders puts additional mechanical stress on the musculature. With regard to structural abnormalities, it should be recognized that there are two types of leg inequality. There is the one which is due to true leg length inequality, and there is the leg length inequality due to spasm of the muscles, particularly the quadratus lumborum muscle. One may be surprised to find that the apparent short leg is in truth the longer leg, but appears to be short because there is spasm of the quadratus muscle on that side. Unawareness of this may result in putting a corrective heel lift in the wrong shoe with the result that you have made the patient worse rather than better.

Fibrositis is another cause of mechanical headache. There are those who do not believe that it is a real entity, but in the clinical opinion of many clinicians it is not only real, but commonplace. Again, in order to identify it, one must use the examining hand rather than rely on a specific laboratory study. There is a great overlap in the group of patients who have fibrositis and those who develop this type of headache. Much of it relates to people with similar personality traits, but the majority of it results from problems in the musculature, leading to the formation of trigger points with their referred pattern of pain.

A discussion of problems in the musculature cannot be complete without a discussion of problems in the joints, since the two are closely related. Variously called the facet syndrome, joint lock, or joint dysfunction, this problem does not produce visible (on x-ray films) joint pathology. Rather, there is a loss of involuntary motion (not under the control of our muscles) which is common to all synovial joints and which provides protection from sudden extremes of motion. Whether the problem is primary, resulting from trauma, disuse, or faulty mechanics, and the lack of motion producing secondary changes in the muscles, or whether the problem in the joints is secondary to changes in the muscles, attention must be paid to both if relief is to be obtained.

Temporomandibular joint problems and related problems of imbalance of the mandible are responsible for both facial pain and headache. It should be remembered, however, that problems here may cause problems in the neck and upper back which, in turn, will be a cause for headache. Finally, we come to the etiologic factor of tension which is a common thread running through most of these patients. Although its importance cannot be denied, it should not blind us to other factors that play their own role in causation.

History-Taking

The principles of history-taking in the headache patient has already been covered elsewhere. However, a few brief points regarding its role in mechanical headache would be in order. It is usually stated that 90% of patients with this type of headache report having bilateral pain. It is usually true that if the pain is bilateral it is posterior in origin. However, if the pains are anterior in origin, the pain may be bilateral, bilateral with unilateral predominance, alternating bilaterally, unilateral or some variation of these.

The character of the pain is usually dull and persistent but may at times be described as sharp and shooting. A band-like feeling is often described and words like aching, tightness, heaviness, and pressure are often used. Sleep disturbance is frequent, as is awakening in the morning with a headache present. Major social disturbances can often be gleaned from the history, and one is struck by the lack of insight shown by the patient as to his own makeup playing a role in causation of the problem. Anxiety and depression are often written on the faces of these patients, but this is true of most chronic pain patients and it is difficult to separate cause and effect.

It should be asked whether there is any increased symptomatology with change of barometric pressure. We do know that it is more than just an old wives' tale, that patients with joint problems can anticipate change in barometric pressure; however, it is equally true that patients with muscle problems can do the same thing. Questions should be raised about the presence of jaw pain or crepitus on chewing, change in bite, and the presence of bruxism at night. It is also important to inquire about the type of work performed by the patient and whether or not there are any difficulties in the remainder of the spine.

Physical Examination

In examining the patient with this type of headache, one has to examine the entire spine and, therefore, the patient has to be undressed. One looks at the posture which is exhibited, ie, the spinal curves, the slope of the shoulders, and the size of the breasts all are factors in the production of headache. It is important to observe the height of the pelvic crest in order to determine leg length inequality. The usual method for determining leg length inequality is to measure from the anterior superior iliac spine to the medial malleolus. This is grossly inaccurate; if you do three measurements you often obtain three completely different answers, particularly in an obese person in whom the difficulty is in finding the anterior superior iliac spine in the first place. Therefore, there are three ways that one can examine for pelvic obliquity: "eyeball it" at the level of the pelvic crest, observe the level of the posterior superior iliac spines, and observe the level of the parasacral dimples. Often one cannot see the posterior iliac spines or the parasacral dimples; therefore, the best way is to observe any inequality in the heights of the pelvic crest.

Tightness of the lumbodorsal fascia, the thoracodorsal, and cervical fascia, and tightness of all the posterior musculature including the neck and back muscles, the quadratus lumborum muscles, the gluteal musculature, and the hamstring muscles must be assessed.

Careful palpation of the suboccipital musculature in the supine position will reveal spasm of these muscles. Often, pressure here will reproduce the headache and raise the question of entrapment of the great occipital nerve. However, trigger points in the muscles or joint dysfunction in the upper cervical facet joints may be equally at fault.

Range of motion of the entire spine but most particularly the cervical spine must be looked for. A goniometer is helpful in recording the motion since it is important to have an objective number to compare before and after treatment. If the values are clearly improving, no matter what the complaints of the patients, one can feel comfortable in that one is making progress with the treatment.

Examination of the face should include careful palpation of the temporal arteries. In addition, a basic examination of the TMJ and its surrounding structures should include observation of the bite (underbite, overbite), the opening of the jaw (symmetrical or asymmetrical), and the size of the aperture (roughly measured by the number of knuckles that can be admitted). Palpation of the TMJ for tenderness as well as palpation of the surrounding musculature is next, followed by evaluation of condylar position and crepitus by having the patient open and close the jaws with the examiner's little fingers in the patient's ear. Normally, the condyles are not palpable with this maneuver and crepitus cannot be felt.

One must look for trigger points and the jump signs that were described. It is important to perform the skin rolling maneuver which is always positive in fibrositis. Here, one picks up the skin of the back and rolls between thumb and forefinger. Normally, tissues glide one over the other with a mild pinching sensation or a slight discomfort being felt by the patient. Those who have fibrositis have adherence of all the layers: skin on subcutaneous tissue, subcutaneous tissue on fascia, and fascia on muscle, and, therefore, skin rolling demonstrates tightness and produces tenderness and pain. This has to be corrected as part of the treatment program. With the patient in the supine position so that the muscles are relaxed, one can carefully palpate the suboccipital musculature for observation of local tightness or tenderness and palpate over the cervical neural foramina to see if there is any evidence of synovitis of the joint, or if there is any tenderness of the overlying ligaments. If the former exists, the tenderness will be localized to one neural foramina; in the latter, there will be diffuse tenderness. By examining for this in the supine position with the neck muscles relaxed, the examining fingers fall right into the neural foramina.

Treatment

The goals of treatment are twofold, alteration of the pathologic changes and prevention of future problems. Drug therapy can be described as being only moderately effective, its principal role being that of an adjuvant or for use as a maintenance treatment. There are five classes of drugs used in treating these types of problems:

1. Muscle relaxants
2. Anti-inflammatory agents
3. Analgesics
4. Sedatives and hypnotics
5. Antidepressants and antianxiety agents

Although muscle relaxants are used, their efficacy or worth is uncertain and they probably function as central nervous system sedatives. The anti-inflammatory medications are useful, the drugs in question being the nonsteroidal anti-inflammatory drugs. The reason for their usefulness is uncertain but there may well be a low-grade sterile inflammation in some of these trigger points. If the problem is that of myofascial pain or fibrositis, this class of drugs is often quite helpful, particularly during therapy when there is usually a flare-up of pain. Some of the newer analgesics (zomepirac sodium or naproxen sodium) are derivatives of a nonsteroidal anti-inflammatory agent and share both characteristics. The use of analgesics is obvious, with the least amount and the least addicting medications being the best. Although a wide range of sedatives and hypnotic drugs are available, a combination of a barbiturate with either an aspirin phenacetin and caffeine combination or with acetaminophen appear to be particularly effective in this type of headache. Antidepressant medications are most effective in those depressed patients who have difficulty sleeping and awake in the morning with headache as severe as upon going to sleep. Use of drugs such as amitriptyline or doxepin taken in a single dosage at bedtime may markedly improve sleep and relieve depression throughout the day, without producing daytime lethargy. For those patients in whom anxiety or related states may predominate, the use of a phenothiazine drug such as fluphenazine may be helpful.

If mechanical problems exist, they have to be corrected. If there is a true pelvic obliquity (one not due to spasm of the spine muscles), it is helpful to correct this obliquity with heel lifts for reasons mentioned before. The simplest way to do that is by means of trial and error, using a series of blocks to find out what is most comfortable for the patient. Temporary heel lifts which are transferred to all of the patient's footwear are used as a trial and if, after a period of time has elapsed this proves to be beneficial, then permanent lifts are prescribed. If, on the other hand, the pelvic obliquity is due to muscle spasm, then this too must be corrected. Posture and body mechanics are most important to work with. Proper bras for the patient with large breasts might include a longline bra, wire under the bra, broad shoulder straps, and padding under the shoulder straps. Reduction mammoplasty might be considered in rare cases. Appropriate alteration of work habits may be helpful, although there is no need to make a fetish of altering work habits unless there is something obvious which needs to be altered.

Physical therapy techniques are very helpful in the treatment of soft tissue problems. There are two things to be aware of in prescribing the treatment. First, the treatment should be directed to the pathology, and, second, the treatment program should be modified as the pathology changes. Ordering heat and massage ad infinitum when the pathologic condition requires that an appropriate corrective exercise program is indicated benefits nobody. If the problem is degenerative joint disease with asynovitis of the joints, pulsed ultrasound is helpful. One can obtain a very high wattage from using the pulsed mode, and since one of the effects of ultrasound is to increase the permeability of semipermeable membranes (and the synovial lining of the joint is a semipermeable membrane), one can help to reduce the edema and swelling about the joint. Iontophoresis may be used in the same fashion. If the muscles are tight or tender, they have trigger points and these must be removed; restoration of normal range of motion is essential. If the problem is fibrositis, one must treat the muscles as mentioned before by restoring the normal gliding motion. This is performed by using the skin rolling techniques, not as a diagnostic test but as a therapeutic tool.

Painful trigger points causing or contributing to headache have to be abolished. The initial treatment is the use of physical therapy modalities. The most common ones that we use are ultrasound combined with electrical stimulation, the vapocoolant spray (using a fluorimethane vapor as popularized by Dr. Janet Travell), and the high-voltage galvanic current. They all have a common rationale in providing a barrage of afferent stimuli into the spinal cord, which alters the perception of pain. This must then be followed by stretching and eventually strengthening of the affected muscles. If the suboccipital muscles are part of the pattern, it is important that suboccipital massage be utilized. If tightness is part of the problem and is in the atlanto-occipital joints, either primary or secondary because of spasm of the suboccipital muscles, this then must be relieved by manipulative technique.

If these physical therapy techniques are not completely effective, they are supplemented with injections which have the same rationale as the physical modalities in that they provide a barrage of afferent impulses which temporarily block the pain pattern, permitting efforts to be directed to the restoration of normal motion. Initial treatment is with 0.5% bupivacaine, and the injection is performed with a very finely gauged needle directed into the trigger point. It is interesting to note that initially in patients with very active trigger points, one can locate without great difficulty the trigger point. Upon location of the trigger point the affected segment of the muscle fasciculates. This is encouraging because you know that you are in the area of pathology and that you have injected the medication in an appropriate place. Normal muscle is insensitive and does not fasciculate when touched by the probing needle. Upon touching the trigger point, the patient often notes that the pain is in the same distribution of which he has been complaining. If there is a favorable response to the bupivacaine injection which lasts without recurrences, nothing further is done. If there is a temporary response, then steroids may be added to the solution. Their benefit would seem to be suppression of the low-grade inflammatory response previously mentioned. In a rare patient who is sensitive to bupivacaine or to lidocaine, then sterile saline can be substituted. Often a series of injections is necessary.

It needs to be emphasized that all of the above is preliminary to adequate stretching of the muscle. This is performed by the therapist but must be followed through by a home program on the part of the patient. Multiple brief stretchings throughout the day are preferable to a single exercise session and the patient must be instructed to do the stretching *through* the point of pain and not just *to* the point of pain. As spasms ease, strengthening exercises are added, usually in the form of isometric exercises. Again, multiple brief sessions throughout the day are encouraged.

Problems in the facet joints of the cervical and thoracic spine may have to be relieved by manipulative techniques. These can be considered to be simply another modality of treatment. They can be detected only with the proper examining maneuvers and relieved with the proper techniques, which are detailed in the accompanying bibliography.

In addition to all of the above, attention must be directed to relief of tension. There is often little insight on the part of the patient as to the role this is playing in the perpetuation of the headache. Conversely, many patients are told that "it is all in their head" and they are unable to understand how they can hurt so much if that is so. Therefore, an explanation which includes the role of tension, presence of organicity in the musculoskeletal structures, the ability to treat the problem but the likelihood of relapses, and the absence of a "magic bullet" to cure it instantly help the patient be a participant in the treatment process.

Relief of tension may be carried out in several ways. Handing the patient a prescription for an antianxiety or antidepressant medication is the least effective. Autogenic (self) training is useful, and this may be done by the use of Jacobson's relaxation exercises or by use of a relaxation tape. Other autogenic techniques include yoga or transcendental meditation; some patients may benefit from being trained in self-hypnosis.

Autogenic training can be augmented where necessary by the use of biofeedback techniques. Electromyographic biofeedback is a technique for control of the muscles in which the patient is placed in a closed loop system with the machine; the patient can voluntarily alter the output (sound, digital readout, wave form) by tensing or relaxing his muscles. By obtaining immediate feedback on the state of the muscle tension, the patient is able to train himself to alter this tension. The early settings are made easily but as the training sessions progress, the instructor makes them progressively more difficult. In the use of this technique for the treatment of patients with headache, muscles are often chosen because they are readily accessible. The frontalis muscle is one frequently picked. It is far more effective, however, to identify the painful muscles in spasm and to select these muscles for treatment.

Many patients respond to these techniques and the sympathetic ear of the physician. For those who do not, psychotherapy becomes a necessary adjunct to treatment.

It is clear that this problem is difficult and troubling to treat. As in most chronic pain problems, adaptation to the pain is often the only goal left to the treating physician, and this is certainly a worthwhile goal in itself. This may be accomplished by individual treatment and counseling or by a group treatment program as offered by many pain clinics. However, for many other patients, employing the techniques mentioned above, permanent or marked relief may be obtained.

BIBLIOGRAPHY

Bonica JJ: Management of myofascial pain syndromes in general practice. *JAMA* 1957;164:732.

Brown Burnell R Jr: Diagnosis and therapy of common myofascial syndromes. *JAMA* 1978;239:7.

Fowler RS, Kraft GH: Tension perception in patients having pain associated with chronic muscle tension. *Arch Phys Med Rehabil* 1974;55:28.

Grant AE: Massage with ice (cyrokinetics) and treatment of pain conditions of the musculoskeletal system. *Arch Phys Med Rehabil* 1964;45:233.

Jacobsen E: *Progressive Relaxation.* Chicago, University of Chicago Press, 1938.

Kapandji IA: *The Physiology of the Joints,* ed 2. London, Churchill Livingston, vol 3, 1974.

Melzack R, Wall PD: Pain mechanisms: A new theory. *Science* 1965;150:971.

Mennell JMcM: *Back Pain.* Boston, Little, Brown and Company, 1960.

Travell JG, Rinzler SH: The myofascial genesis of pain. *Postgrad Med* 1952;11:425.

Zohn DA, Mennell JMcM: *Musculoskeletal Pain: Diagnosis and Physical Treatment.* Boston, Little, Brown and Company, 1976.

Zohn DA: Pain caused by large breasts. *Human Sexuality* August, 1979.

12 Surgical Evaluation and Treatment of Headache

Donlin M. Long

A large number of operations are done for the complaint of headaches which are difficult to justify from the data reported in the literature. However, there are important surgical aspects of the headache problem that requires some discussion. The first part of this chapter deals with the diagnosis, that is, when to suspect that a patient who comes into an office complaining of a headache has an underlying neurosurgical problem that requires therapy. The second part deals with the surgical therapy of the very small number of highly specific headache problems.

Headache as a Neurological Complaint

When is it appropriate to mount a full-scale neurological evaluation for a patient presenting with the complaint of headache? It is well-known that headache is the most common symptom of a patient with a brain tumor; 75% of patients with brain tumors complain of headache.

However, of the patients who have headaches, an extremely small percentage will eventually be found to have brain tumors. It is estimated that there are 25,000,000 people with headaches in the United States, and there are probably 10,000 newly discovered primary brain tumors each year.

There are some specific situations which suggest and even demand further investigation. First is the coincidental occurrence of any other neurological symptoms. In the case of headaches due to brain tumors, the most common accompanying symptom is seizures. The combination of chronic headache and an epileptic seizure is highly suspicious for tumor, and should always be investigated. This underscores the observation that most patients with headaches do not develop neurological deficits at any point in their symptomatology in the absence of a structural lesion. Of course, there always are exceptions, but the rule is a safe one. When there are other neurological findings, it is possible that there is an underlying tumor. Any kind of brain tumor can cause headache, but, characteristically, posterior fossa tumors produce hydrocephalus and cause significant headache. Headache in a child is a much more specific symptom of brain tumor than headache in an adult. An unusually persisting headache in a child needs an evaluation for a posterior fossa tumor.

The second factor that is highly suggestive of a tumor is a postural variation in the headache. A typical example was recently seen on the neurological service at Johns Hopkins Hospital. A 43-year-old woman, who had been evaluated for seven years for the complaint of facial pain, was admitted for neurosurgical evaluation. She complained of pain behind the eye. When she put her head down between her knees, her headache disappeared. However, when she sat upright, this created headache pain. One can visualize a flap of tumor tissue in the third ventricle that would block the outflow of cerebral spinal fluid when the patient was erect, thereby causing the headache; the same flap of tissue would fall forward when the patient bent her head between her knees, allowing the appropriate flow of cerebral spinal fluid. This is the classic "ball valve" action of an intraventricular tumor. The computed tomographic (CT) scan showed a large, benign ventricular tumor which was removed, and her pain disappeared.

There is another group of individuals with arrested hydrocephalus who sometimes will develop headache mimicing tumor. The important aspect of the history is the report of a large head early in life, which stopped growing with or without therapy. Typically, the head size will be in the upper range of normal variation, and the child or adult will complain of chronic headaches. Very often, arrested hydrocephalus is not really arrested and will become active at some point in late childhood to early adult life. As the pressure slowly increases and the flow of cerebral spinal fluid is impeded, the headache becomes a more important symptom. This diagnosis is easily made because of the evidence of large head size and the antecedent history. CT scan is the confirmatory diagnostic test.

Another neurological condition associated with headache is an aneurysm. These outpouchings of cerebral arteries occasionally will present with headaches. The unusual presentation consists of generalized headache, present throughout the entire head, related to a warning leak. The patient with specific pain in the eye occasionally will have an aneurysm, typically of the carotid artery. The pain may occur by two mechanisms. There may be pressure on the undersurface of the tentorium. The aneurysms that are usually associated with face pain and headache are large aneurysms of the carotid artery. As the aneurysm enlarges, tentorial pressure produces pain in the face, usually in the distribution of the first and second division of the trigeminal nerve (fifth nerve) which radiates into the eye and to the cheek. Aneurysms may also produce a third-nerve palsy associated with the facial pain in the same distribution. While the palsy may not be complete, there will be a deficit in pupillary reaction. The pupil is usually slightly enlarged and does not react well to light; on careful examination one will also detect a sensory loss in the trigeminal division. When the patient develops both third-nerve and fifth-nerve neurological deficits, one should be suspicious of an aneurysm of the cavernous sinus causing the eye pain by direct nerve compression.

Tumors at the base of the skull also cause pain. It is usually very severe and has the unremitting character of cancer pain. There are two important factors to consider. The first is the history of having a persistent characteristic intractable pain. The other factor is that the pain may occur long before bony destruction at the base of the skull is evident on skull x-ray films. It is always important to remember this whenever the head pain is suspected to be due to cancer.

These tumors consist of two types. The first involves the trigeminal ganglion at the base of the temporal lobe. These may be malignant neurofibromas, occasionally menigiomas, or simple neurofibromas of the Gasserian ganglion. The pain is in the distribution of the trigeminal nerve, radiating into the face. Unlike trigeminal neuralgia, the pain associated with tumors of the trigeminal ganglion is constant and not episodic.

The second type of facial pain due to cancer is associated with a paranasal sinus carcinoma. On occasion, these carcinomas may invade the base of the skull and when this occurs, the pain has the same characteristic, unremitting nature. It is also deep-seated and is reported to be associated with sinus pain. Diagnosis of both is normally made by skull roentgenograms which show the bony erosion due to the tumor. It is also essential to conduct a thorough ear, nose, and throat examination and a careful sensory evaluation. CT scan of the skull is of great value. Unfortunately, before bony destruction occurs the diagnosis can be extremely difficult to establish.

The final diagnostic category that falls in the area of neurosurgical face and head pain are lesions of the cervical spine. There are several important types. Atlanto-axial dislocations, usually congenital in type, are brought about by some later trauma at which time the underlying deficit is discovered. Basilar impression and the Arnold-Chiari malformation may both require surgical intervention. Usually, the congenital anomalies are easy to diagnose. Headache is not as important a symptom as is neck pain, with radiation into the suboccipital region. The Arnold-Chiari malformation is an exception. This is a congenital anomaly of the hind brain in which the outflow of cerebral spinal fluid from the fourth ventricle is blocked. Very often, there may be hydrocephalus present and the earliest complaint is headache. This is present before neurological deficit occurs. For reasons which are unclear, simple decompression consisting of removal of the bony compression of the cervical medullary junction is usually adequate to relieve the headache. Sometimes the hydrocephalus is severe, and a shunt is required. However, the headache often is apparently related to the bony compression at the base of the skull. Logue utilizes a simple surgical procedure which removes the posterior occipital bone and the arch of C-1 and C-2, decompressing the upper cervical spine and the upper cervical nerve roots (specifically C-1, C-2, and C-3). Relieving pressure due to bony compression of the cerebellum and midbrain, this procedure usually results in excellent control of headache. In most of these cases, there are progressive neurological deficits related to medullary and upper spinal cord compression, which are treated by intradural decompression.

The most controversial headache problems often managed by surgery are those that relate to cervical disc degeneration and cervical spondylosis. Many of the anterior cervical fusions done in the United States are apparently done for the complaint of neck pain and headache, not for complaints of radicular compression. There is a great deal of disagreement between neurosurgeons which is focused on the validity of this technique for neck pain and headache, but the best data in the literature indicate that the relief of headache and neck pain by intercervical fusion is minimal at best.

Appropriate Selection of Diagnostic Tests

One question that always arises is when to obtain a CT scan in the evaluation of a patient with a headache. It is more appropriate to ask, "When is it appropriate to evaluate headache with adjunctive tests?" Skull x-ray films are routine except in those headache syndromes which are absolutely typical, ie, the migraine and its variants and cluster headache. In these cases, it may be more appropriate to evaluate a patient's response to medical management rather than obtaining a battery of tests. Therapy of migrainous headaches is discussed in Chapter 13 as is treatment of myofascial disorders, which are discussed in Chapters 11, 14, 15, and 22. However, if there is any variation from typical syndromes, then plain skull films are certainly appropriate. The electroencephalogram (EEG) may be of some use if the headaches are episodic in nature, or if there is any neurological reason to obtain this test. It is not feasible to perform 25,000,000 CT scans to screen every patient who complains of headache; this test should be limited only to patients with an atypical history, an associated neurological deficit, or failure to respond to therapy. Even then, the majority of CT scans will be normal, but it is reasonable to perform this diagnostic test when there is no response to adequate therapy. The newer CT scan techniques showing bony detail will supplant skull x-ray films in the diagnosis of headache. Echoencephalography, radionuclide scans, and pneumoencephalograms have been eliminated from headache evaluation by CT scans.

Surgical Procedures for Symptomatic Relief of Headache

The most common operation for headache is sectioning the greater occipital nerve. The greater occipital nerves are sectioned where they penetrate the muscular layer; this is done through a small transverse incision usually under local anesthesia. This procedure is done for the typical "muscle tension headache," when it is localized in the occipital region, with radiations to the top of the skull. It is called "greater occipital neuralgia," which is a descriptive term that has some degree of validity. However, these are usually tension headaches generated by nerve compression in the cervical musculature. If a peripheral block is done using 1% Xylocaine, most of these patients will be relieved. If Xylocaine is ineffective, then the addition of 20 mg of Depo Medrol with 2 to 3 ml of 1% Xylocaine in the occipital nerve area may be an effective therapy. If the patient does have a positive response to Xylocaine and Xylocaine with Depo Medrol but the effect is not permanent, then one may consider occipital nerve sectioning. Patients who fail to respond to Xylocaine blocks are obviously not candidates for sectioning of the occipital nerve.

If the patient obtains repeated relief with nerve blocks and one does not wish to pursue a surgical intervention, there is an alternative approach. Instead of actually cutting the nerve, it is identified by palpation, and a stimulating electrode is placed in the canal percutaneously under a local anesthesia. Stimulation is continued until there is sensation in the distribution of the greater occipital nerve over the top of the head; then, a differential heat lesion is performed in which one attempts to destroy the pain-carrying fibers without making the back of the head totally anesthetic. This is a very important point, since many patients who have experienced an anesthesia over the occiput find this unpleasant. They report that they cannot tell the location of their head on the pillow, they cannot tell when the head touches something when they lean back, and they are not very pleased even if their headache is improved. Utilizing the differential heat technique, it is possible to produce analgesia and hypesthesia without total anesthesia. Unfortunately, the technique is not as exact as with the differential thermocoagulation of the Gasserian ganglion for trigeminal neuralgia.

The second headache where the neurosurgeon may provide some benefit for the patient is in the treatment of temporal arteritis or an occasional unusual migraine syndrome. Usually, the neurosurgeon will receive a request to do a biopsy in a vascular headache syndrome in order to diagnose the temporal arteritis syndrome. Occasionally, these patients actually will improve due to the surgery alone. Unfortunately, there are no clear-cut criteria to differentiate between the patients who will have direct benefit from a temporal-artery biopsy, as opposed to those patients who do not, so one must view any improvement as a bonus. In no instance should temporal-artery biopsy be considered a treatment of choice or a cure, and temporal arteritis must be treated with steroids, even if headache is relieved.

The only major new development concerning surgical therapy of headache is the microvascular decompression popularized by Janetta. Interestingly, in the 1920s, Walter Dandy of Johns Hopkins Hospital felt that trigeminal neuralgia and many other kinds of facial and ear pains were caused by compression of the trigeminal nerve (fifth cranial nerve) in the posterior fossa, usually by a vascular loop and sometimes by tumor. Janetta began treating trigeminal neuralgia by removing the vascular loops from the fifth nerve, and reported in a short-term follow-up study of 50 patients that 96% were completely relieved of their trigeminal neuralgia. The general success rates are in the range of 80%. The concept of vascular loop compression can be applied to a variety of cranial nerve syndromes. Branches of the anterior-inferior cerebellar artery have been found to compress to nervus intermedius and the seventh and eighth cranial nerves which can produce tinnitus, vertigo, and hemifacial spasm. Additionally, loops of the anterior-inferior cerebral artery may also compress the ninth and tenth cranial nerves and cause pharyngeal neuralgia.

The operation for trigeminal neuralgia is designed to dissect blood vessels free from the brainstem and the particular cranial nerve. A small pledget holds the vessel away from the nerve which is ostensibly being compressed. For patients with trigeminal neuralgia, utilizing this technique, Janetta has reported 80+ % of the patients obtained relief. Additionally, he reports that the majority of patients with classical glossopharyngeal neuralgia were relieved. A small number of patients with classical occipital neuralgia apparently secondary to compression of the second cervical root had been relieved, but the number is too small to make a definitive statement. From the standpoint of headache, the group that is most interesting is the one which falls into two categories: those with cluster headaches of typical nature, and those with atypical facial pain, ie, pain in the face or the head which doesn't fit any clear-cut group. Janetta states that the latter group have trigeminal neuralgia and that they can be relieved by microvascular decompression. He has reported on a few patients with typical cluster headache who did receive relief with microvascular decompression.

These techniques provide an exciting potential for surgery in the area of head and face pain. Although the pain described is not typical headache, it is the kind of pain that one frequently sees in an office practice. Unfortunately, as yet there are no conclusive data concerning the validity of these techniques. Only time and careful follow-up studies of patients will answer whether or not these procedures are applicable beyond typical trigeminal neuralgia. It is difficult to find patients with so-called atypical facial pain who are appropriate candidates for surgery or microvascular dissection because many have associated psychosocial factors.

The author has presented a thumbnail sketch of surgical procedures for headache and face pain. Most of the data in the literature is inconclusive. Some procedures, such as the greater occipital neurectomy, may be overutilized, although there is a place for this type of procedure which may be very useful in carefully selected cases. From the literature, it seems that anterior cervical fusion for the complaint of headache alone is rarely warranted, although clearly some cases are helped. Although the concept of microvascular decompression is most exciting, there are not adequate data at this time that allow one to make a conclusive statement. Beyond the limited applications mentioned, surgery has little use in the therapy of headache.

BIBLIOGRAPHY

Gardner WJ, Stowell A, Dutlinger R: Resection of the greater superficial petrosal nerve in the treatment of unilateral headache. *J Neurosurg* 1947;4:105.

Janetta PJ, Zorub DS: Microvascular decompression for trigeminal neuralgia, in Bucheit W, Truex RC (eds): *Surgery of the Posterior Fossa*. New York, Raven Press, 1979.

Kunkle EC, Wolff HG: Headache, in Baker AB (ed): *Clinical Neurology*. New York, Hoeber-Harper, 1974, vol 2, pp 666–699.

Long DM: Surgical therapy of chronic pain. *Neurosurgery* 1980;6:317.

Olivecrona H: Notes on the surgical treatment of migraine. *Acta Med Scand* 1947; suppl 196.

Wolff H: *Headache and other Head Pain*. New York, Oxford University Press, 1948.

13 Headaches

William G. Speed

One can simplify the classification of headache by considering them under three major categories: 1) vascular, 2) muscle contraction, and 3) traction and inflammatory (Table 13-1). More than 90% of headaches are vascular, muscle contraction, or a combination of the two. Only the most commonly seen headache disorders will be discussed in this chapter.

The clinician who diagnoses and treats headache should take a careful headache history. The pattern of headache serves as the basis for categorizing most headaches. How many types of headaches does the patient have? If there is more than one, then the pattern for each type must be determined separately. Next, determine the age at which headaches were first experienced. What is the frequency of headaches? It is helpful to learn the least frequent rate and the most frequent rate. Averages have little meaning. What is the longest duration of individual attacks of headaches? Next, determine the locations of the headache. Are they ever unilateral? Always? Sometimes? Never? Ask the patient to describe the variations and locations experienced in recurring attacks. What is the

Table 13-1
Headache Classification

Vascular	Muscle Contraction	Traction and Inflammatory
Migraine	Episodic or chronic	Mass lesions (tumors,
Classic		hematoma, aneurysms)
Common	Anxiety and depression	
Hemaplegic		Cranial arteritis
Ophthalmoplegic	TMJ disorder	
Traumatic		Infection
	Cervical degenerative	
Cluster	arteritis	Diseases of EENTT
Episodic		
Chronic	Posttraumatic (some)	Cranial neuralgias
Toxic (pyrexia, pharmacologic, eg, alcohol, CO, nitrates, nitrites)		
Tension (some)		
Posttraumatic (many)		
Hypertension		

range of severity? The author uses a simple, four-level scale to ascertain the range of severity.

1. Level 1, mild and annoying
2. Level 2, moderate
3. Level 3, severe but patient still able to function
4. Level 4, severe and patient no longer able to function

Some patients may experience headaches ranging through all four levels at one time or another, or all headaches may be limited to one or two levels.

It is important to determine the association of headaches with neurologic symptoms such as flashing lights, blurred vision, difficulty in speech, weakness, numbness, tingling in the face, arms, legs, loss of depth perception, vertigo, ataxia, impairment of thought processes, or impairment or loss of consciousness. Inquiry should be made about other associated symptoms, eg, nausea, vomiting, lacrimation, rhinorrhea, and conjunctival infection. The patient should be questioned about headache in other family members.

As many headaches may be influenced by emotional state, the examiner should learn something about the emotional makeup of the patient. The patient should be asked if he considers himself a tense or nervous person and whether there are episodes of feeling tense, irritable, difficulty in relaxing, shaking or sweating of the hands, a lump in the throat, or a knot in the epigastrium, all of which suggest anxiety. One should also inquire about the occurrence of depression and specifically its frequency, duration, and severity. Marked degrees of depression may act as powerful trigger mechanisms for some headache. Is the patient a perfectionist or a chronic worrier? Is there unexplained fatigue? Inquire about sleep patterns. Patients who have difficulty falling asleep are frequently anxious and tense; those who wake up after a few hours and have difficulty getting back to sleep or wake up earlier than their usual time are frequently depressed.

Finally, a careful history of present and past medications for headache should be obtained. Determine what effect, if any, these medications had on the headaches and what side effects have been experienced. Inquire what tests have been carried out in the past and what the results were, and also what consultants, if any, have been seen and what the resultant findings were.

MIGRAINE

Approximately 12 to 15 million people in the United States have migraine, and many of them will ultimately seek help from physicians. Migraine is a constitutional, genetically determined, and psychologically influenced recurrent disorder of the cranial vasculature, the basis of which is a profound instability of cranial vascular regulation. The symptoms range from a mild headache easily tolerated or controlled by simple analgesics to disabling, excruciating, and totally incapacitating headache. Frequently, there is nausea and vomiting, and, in some patients, there may be transient neurological deficits such as impairment of vision, dysarthria, dysphasia, loss of depth perception, vertigo, ataxia, hemiparesis, hemianesthesia, impaired thought processes, impairment of consciousness, or unconsciousness.

The vascular phases of migraine are excessive vasoconstriction and vasodilatation; these two phases may not be sharply separated.

There are many nonspecific migraine-precipitating factors. These are:

1. Psychological triggers (anxiety, depression, etc)
2. Chemical substances (eg, tyramine, phenylethlamine, monosodium glutamate, nitrates and nitrites)
3. Medications (eg, reserpine, nitroglycerin)
4. Meteorologic conditions (eg, low barometric pressure, cold weather, smog)
5. Menstruation
6. Oral contraceptives
7. Exertion
8. Odors (eg, perfumes, exhaust emissions, cigarette smoke, paints, etc)

There is no evidence to indicate that migraine is a primary psychological disorder, but the cranial vascular instability is, of course, vulnerable to emotional stress mechanisms.

Clinical Features

Frequency of migraine attacks may vary from as few as one or two a year to as many as four or five or more per week. Some clinicians believe that they may occur as often as daily, although there is no universal agreement about this among headache specialists. The attacks may last a few hours to several days and sometimes longer, and the intensity varies anywhere from mild to severe and incapacitating. Although the headaches most often occur in the temporal frontal ocular area, they may involve any area of the head or face, alone or in multiple combinations, or they may include the entire head, face, and neck. Often, they are unilateral, and some patients experience unilateral headaches in some attacks and bilateral headaches in others. Yet, other patients have only bilateral headaches. The pains are commonly described as aching, pounding, and throbbing, and are frequently aggravated by jarring the head, bending over, coughing, sneezing, straining, exposure to bright lights, loud noises, and physical exertion. Attacks may begin in early childhood but most often start around puberty or menarche, or perhaps as late as the age of 40.

Management

The management of migraine can be divided into two parts—treatment of acute attacks and prophylaxis.

Treatment of the acute attack Ergotamine tartrate is the treatment of choice for the acute attack. It may be given orally, sublingually, by oral inhalation, rectally, or subcutaneously. Oral preparations are available as Cafergot, Wigraine, and Migral. These are best given as two tablets immediately at the onset of the headache, then two tablets every half hour thereafter until relief, but no more than six tablets per day, and probably no more than ten tablets per week. However, physicians who are thoroughly familiar with the pharmacology of ergotamine and its clinical effects may permit some patients to exceed this total amount per week, provided these patients are under very careful supervision. The tolerance of patients to ergotamine is variable.

Suppositories of Cafergot may be given once rectally immediately at the onset of a headache, repeating once in one hour, if needed, with a maximum of two per day and four per week.

Sublingual tablets (Ergomar, Ergostat) containing 2 mg of ergotamine tartrate may be given as one tablet dissolved under the tongue at the onset of a headache, one tablet repeated at half-hour intervals until relief, and no more than three tablets per day or five tablets per week. Oral inhalations of ergotamine (Riker's Medihaler Ergotamine) may be given as one inhalation immediately at the onset of a headache, repeating one inhalation every five minutes until relief, but not more than six inhalations per day or ten inhalations per week.

Dihydroergotamine mesylate, an ergotamine preparation for subcutaneous use, may be given as 1 ml subcutaneously at the onset of a headache, repeating 1 ml in one hour, if needed, to a maximum of 2 ml per day and 4 ml per week.

Ergotamine compounds should be taken immediately at the onset of a headache. Delay may permit edema to accumulate in the vessel walls, and this effect decreases the ability of ergotamine to exert its vasoconstrictive effect. Prolonged or excessive use of ergotamine compounds may lead to a paradoxical increase in the frequency and duration of headaches. This is apparently related to a state of vascular dependence on ergotamine levels. If the ergotamine levels fall, vascular dilatation develops, producing a headache for which the patient again takes ergotamine, thereby producing a vicious cycle of events. The only way out of this dilemma is to withdraw ergotamine completely, despite the exacerbation of headaches which will ensue; the headaches will usually subside in two to four days.

For those patients who do not respond to ergotamine compounds or who develop side effects, Midrin (isometheptene, dichloralphenazone acetaminophen) may be used. This is given as two capsules at the onset of a headache, one every hour thereafter until relief, with a maximum of five per day.

The contraindications to the use of ergotamine are peripheral vascular disease, severe uncontrolled hypertension, ischemic heart disease, sepsis, hyperthyroidism, pregnancy, and renal and hepatic disease. Side effects are nausea, vomiting, myalgia, paresthesias of the extremities, peripheral spasm, angina, and ergot dependency.

Prophylaxis Prophylactic management should begin with a diet restricting the ingestion of vasoactive chemical substances found in certain foods, which are capable of triggering the migraine process in some patients. These foods include alcohol, chocolate, aged cheese, onions, citrus fruits, coffee (including decaffeinated coffee), tea, chicken livers, fermented sausages, bananas, nuts, Chinese foods, yogurt, canned figs, avocados, hot dogs, and bacon. Such a diet should be continued for several months before deciding it is not effective.

The use of birth control pills should be discouraged. These pills may precipitate migraine in the susceptible individual. They can produce the neurologic manifestations in a migraineur which was not present before starting the pill. Most important to physicians, the use of birth control pills may prevent good control of a migraine syndrome, even though the patient is on what might be considered a good management program.

Inderal (propranolol) is useful in the prophylactic management of migraine, since it seems to stabilize craniovascular function. The usual starting dose is 20 mg four times a day, but larger amounts may be required. Inderal should not be used in patients who have a history of asthma, myocardial insufficiency, peripheral vascular insufficiency, Raynaud's phenomenon, or a marked bradycardia.

Tricyclic antidepressant compounds such as Elavil (amitriptyline) or Trofranil (imipramine) are useful in some patients with migraine, whether or not there is an associated depression. These compounds inhibit the membrane pump mechanism responsible for norepinephrine and serotonin reuptake into the adrenergic and serotinergic neurons. This action may potentiate or prolong sympathetic activity and, hence, increase vascular tone, and thereby be useful in the migraine process. The dosage range is from 25 to 150 mg per day. Postural hypotension, weight gain, sleepiness, and fatigue occasionally occur in these patients, and these may necessitate the discontinuance of these medications. Tricyclic compounds and Inderal may be given together, and in some patients this combination is more effective than when either medication is used alone. Postural hypotensive effect of the tricyclic compounds does not appear to be notably potentiated in most patients when Inderal is added although it can occur.

Sansert and Periactin have antiserotonin properties, and, therefore, are useful in migraine. Sansert has a potential for producing fibroproliferated phenomena, eg, retroperitoneal fibrosis, arterial stenosis, endocardial fibrosis, and pulmonary fibrosis. Therefore, it should be used only by physicians familiar with its pharmacology. It should not be given in the presence of heart murmurs, bruits, coronary artery disease, peripheral vascular disease, or pregnancy. Long-term treatment should be avoided, except under careful medical supervision, and it is suggested that the medication be discontinued for one month out of every three to four months. The usual dose of Sansert is 2 mg three times a day, and if no improvement is noted in three weeks it should be discontinued.

Periactin does not have the fibroproliferating effect that is seen with Sansert. It may produce somnolence in a few patients, particularly in those who had this response with other antihistamines, and it may cause weight gain. It should, therefore, be used with caution in those individuals who have an established weight problem. The dose is 4 mg three to four times a day, and if no response is seen in three or four weeks it should be discontinued. If it proves effective, however, it is not necessary to discontinue it at regular intervals, as is suggested when one is using Sansert.

Biofeedback, using both electromyographic (EMG) and hand warming techniques, may be very useful in the prophylactic management of migraine. This form of therapy works best in younger people and in those patients who have the ability to concentrate and have a strong motivation to get well. It is a method by which the brain can be trained to take over some control of an automatic process which the brain does not inherently possess. Approximately 50% to 60% of individuals appropriately chosen to enter such a training program will benefit. Although some patients obtain good control of their migraine using only biofeedback, others require biofeedback and a combination of pharmacotherapeutic agents.

Finally, emotional trigger mechanisms need to be assessed in the migraine management program. For the most part, a compassionate, interested physician who is willing to devote adequate time to a physician-patient relationship can lessen the impact of some of these trigger mechanisms. A few patients with particularly strong emotional triggers may require referral to a psychiatrist.

CHRONIC POSTTRAUMATIC HEADACHE

Almost anyone who injures his head will have pain or tenderness at the site of impact for hours or several days, and then become free of symptoms. However, about 30% of head-injured patients will develop posttraumatic headache, ie, headaches which have persisted for more than two months. These headaches may mimic almost any type of chronic recurring headache. They may be constant or intermittent. They may involve any area of the head, eg, frontal, temporal, vertex, occipital, alone or in any combination, they may be unilateral, bilateral, or generalized, and patients may exhibit more than one type of headache. Pains may be aching, pressing, squeezing, expanding, burning, stabbing, throbbing, or pounding, depending on the specific mechanism involved. The mechanisms involved are muscle contraction, vasodilatation (including the migraine process), scar formation in the scalp, or injuries to neck structures. They may be seen alone or in any combination. Management, of course, depends on the mechanism involved and is discussed elsewhere in this presentation. However, treatment of the so-called "whiplash injury" should be conservative; a cervical collar should be tried along with heat and massage. Occasionally, Xylocaine, with or without cortical steroids, injected into localized tender areas of the neck may be beneficial. However, prolonged disability is not rare.

CLUSTER HEADACHES

This is a much less common variety of vascular headaches than migraine. It is estimated to occur in about 0.5% of the population. It is a male-dominated disorder. It can appear at any age, but most occur between 20 and 40 years of age. The clusters frequently occur in the spring or fall, but are not limited to these times. The cluster durations last for weeks or months, and infrequently may become chronic, lasting for years.

The individual attacks of pain are of short duration, lasting 10 to 120 minutes, rarely longer. One to three attacks per 24 hours are common, many are nocturnal, awakening the patient one to two hours after going to sleep. The remission in between clusters may last for weeks, months, or years. The pain is associated with dilatation of both the external and internal carotid systems. The pain is experienced predominantly in the temporo-ocular-maxillary area or areas. The intensity is usually quite severe, and its peak level is likely to be experienced within a few minutes of the onset. The headaches are burning, boring, gnawing, throbbing, or pounding in nature, essentially are always unilateral, and tend to involve the same side throughout a given cluster. Unilateral rhinorrhea, nasal congestion, and lacrimation of conjunctival injunction frequently accompany the pain. Unilateral, ocular, sympathetic paresis (ptosis and myosis) occurs occasionally, and is usually, but not always, transient. The attacks may be precipitated by the ingestion of alcohol or lying down to take a nap.

Management

A few simple measures are sometimes useful for patients with predominantly nocturnal episodes. Elevating the legs of the head of the bed on 8- to 10-in blocks occasionally prevents the nocturnal attacks. If it does not work within a night or two, there is no need to continue it. Inhalation of oxygen immediately at the onset of a headache at 7 liters/min for 15 min sometimes will abort an attack. Immersing the hands, wrists, and forearms in ice water promptly at the onset of an attack will sometimes shorten them.

Ergotamine tartrate is the treatment of choice. Since many cluster headaches occur at a predicted time, it is possible to give an effective dose shortly before the onset. With appropriate physician supervision, ergotamine tartrate up to 4 mg can be given orally in a 24-hour period. With particularly difficult clusters, the patient can be taught the self-administration of DHE45 subcutaneously. One ml can be given once or twice a day, but careful monitoring of the patient is essential, since the medication is given over a long period of time. It should be emphasized that any physician using ergotamine compounds or any of the pharmacotherapeutic measures used for headache should make him/herself totally knowledgeable concerning the dose, indications, and long-term effects of these medications.

Sansert is sometimes useful. This may be given as 2 mg three times a day. The same cautions previously noted must be observed.

Prednisone may control some cluster headaches, but if beneficial response is not obtained in a two- or three-day period, this medication should be promptly discontinued. Therapy begins with a 60-mg dose per day, with subsequent gradual reduction to a more reasonable maintenance level. Unfortunately, many patients with cluster headaches require rather large doses for control. Therefore, this method of treatment may not be useful from a practical point of view. There are side effects from long-term use of prednisone, such as an increased incidence of cataracts, coronary artery disease, osteoporosis, and asymptomatic necrosis of the hip. Physician judgment, therefore, is important.

Finally, for those patients whose cluster headaches have become chronic, that is, persisting for more than six months without a remission, one may use lithium carbonate. The usual dose is 300 mg three times a day, blood levels should be kept below 1 mEq/liter, and appropriate physician follow up is essential. If good response is not obtained in ten days or two weeks, it should be discontinued. Psychotherapy has no appreciable role in the management of cluster headache patients. Biofeedback has not been proved useful.

MUSCLE CONTRACTION HEADACHES

Muscle contraction headache is a common variety of headache which occurs in two forms, episodic and chronic.

The episodic type is the most common, and most patients with this disorder never seek the services of a physician. The headaches are usually mild to moderate in intensity and involve the vertex or the temporal, frontal, or occipital cervical regions separately or in any combination. Most often, they are described as tight pressure, squeezing, aching, and usually triggered by such things as fatigue, an acute family crisis, or carrying a stressful work load. They usually subside following the cessation of the offending stimulus, or may be relieved by various over-the-counter analgesics.

The chronic variety presents a more difficult management problem. Usually, the pains are constant and unremitting and may be present for weeks, months, years, or decades. The same areas of the head are involved as in the acute type, and the characteristics are similar.

Muscle contraction headaches may be secondary to underlying disorders such as: 1) disturbances of the eye (inflammation, muscle imbalance), 2) nasal or paranasal inflammation, 3) temporomandibular joint dysfunction, 4) disorders of the neck (degenerative arthritis, ankylosing spondylosis, and discogenic disease), 5) inflammation secondary to systemic disorders (viral infections), 6) trauma, including nerve entrapment, 7) high cervical or posterior fossa tumor (slow-growing astrocytoma or meningioma), or 8) vascular headaches. However, most chronic muscle contraction headaches are associated with tension, anxiety, depression, repressed hostility, anger, unresolved dependency needs, or psychosexual conflict. The diagnosis, as in many other headaches, is dependent on the patterns of the headache obtained by a good history.

Management

Treatment of chronic muscle contraction headache consists first of stopping the use of analgesic medication, which so many of these patients take on a regular basis. There is good analgesic medication for recurrent acute pain, but good analgesics for treating chronic, nonterminal pain probably do not exist. There is some suggestion that the long-term use of chronic analgesics may actually perpetuate the chronicity of the pain of chronic muscle contraction headache. Therefore, a strong effort should be exerted by the physician to have patients discontinue this chronic use.

Usually, local heat and massage is of little help. Tricyclic compounds appear to be the most useful of the pharmacological agents available. The dosage is that described for migraine. It is of interest that Inderal is sometimes helpful, although this medication has not been approved by the Food and Drug Administration for headache of this type. It is used frequently in combination with tricyclic compounds. The drug combats the effects of anxiety, which may explain its beneficial response in some instances, but the author believes that the drug's efficacy is related to the associated vascular components of muscle contraction headaches which are not clinically recognized. Tranquilizers are not a great deal of help, but judicious use of phenothiazines such as fluphenazine occasionally may be tried. It is probably best to avoid tranquilizers like diazepam because of their potential for habituation with long-term use, and the possibility of enhancing depression.

Biofeedback is of value for many patients with this disorder. Also, a good physician-patient relationship is important, and repeated office interviews may prove to be rewarding. Physicians must be willing to commit a fair amount of time to working with patients with this problem. It is generally accepted that emotional factors may be a common precipitant for muscle contraction headaches via the translation of anxiety into a physical symptom, or a symbolic communication of psychogenic distress. The genesis of such anxiety may be rooted in the individual's past interpersonal conflicts, and, therefore, some muscle contraction headache patients may require psychiatric referral.

CRANIAL ARTERITIS

Cranial arteritis is a disorder of the older age group. Essentially all patients with this disorder are over the age of 50, and most are over the age of 60. When a headache begins for the first time in someone over the age of 50, or a change of the characteristics of a previously recurring headache occurs in this age group, cranial arteritis should be high on one's list of suspicion. It affects both sexes, women somewhat more than men. It is characterized by painful inflammation of the cranial arteries and associated with general systemic signs and symptoms, eg, malaise, weight loss, fever, sweating, and weakness. Sometimes the symptoms are subtle and the patient's complaints have been mistaken for depression. The sedimentation rate is almost always markedly elevated, and there may be mild to moderate elevation of the leukocyte count. Pathologically, there is a giant cell arteritis, which probably represents a disorder of immunologic vasculitis associated with the deposition of immune complexes within the walls of the involved arteries.

The headache is nonspecific and is likely to be diffuse or generalized, but may be localized to the regions along the arteries of the scalp. It is often aching, throbbing, or burning, and varies from moderate to severe in intensity. The scalp is frequently tender to touch, particularly along the arteries. Pulsation of the arteries may or may not be absent. Intermittent claudication of the jaws sometimes occurs.

The most dreaded complication of this disorder is blindness resulting from arteritis of the ophthalmic artery, and subsequent optic ischemia appears. This complication can usually be avoided by the early institution of adrenal cortical steriod therapy, eg, prednisone 60 mg a day, or its equivalent, to start. Reasonable suspicion of the diagnosis is sufficient in most cases to begin prednisone therapy promptly. If the diagnosis is correct, prompt resolution of the headache can sometimes occur in 24 to 72 hours—one of the most dramatic symptom responses seen in any medical disorder. If response does not occur within 72 hours, then the diagnosis should be reassessed.

The diagnosis can usually be established by a biopsy of the involved artery; however a negative biopsy does not exclude the diagnosis. The arterial lesions may "skip"; hence, a large segment of artery should be removed and a diligent search made by the pathologist. Prednisone should be gradually reduced over a period of weeks or months at a rate determined by symptoms and the sedimentation rate. A maintenance dose may be required for weeks, months, or, more usually, years. Basically, it appears to be a self-limiting disorder, and eventually prednisone can be stopped in most patients.

COMMENTS

The author has tried to describe some of the more important and common headaches which may be a problem to clinicians in an office practice. Certain symptoms represent alarm of warning signals. Sudden, severe headache raises the suspicion of a subdural hemorrhage. Severe headaches associated with fever are seen with various viral syndromes, but one has to be certain that one is not dealing with meningitis or encephalitis. Obviously, an adequate history and a physical examination will make this differentiation. Headaches associated with convulsion suggest an organic intracranial abnormality. Although headaches accompanied by confusion or decreasing consciousness may be associated with the migraine process, if they have not represented a previous pattern with headache, then an intracranial organic abnormality may be present. Most patients with a blow to the head will have headache but will not have any demonstrable medical or structural abnormalities. However, the possibility of more serious disorders, such as subdural hematoma and ETC, must be kept in mind. Headache with localized eye pain may represent migraine or glaucoma. The latter diagnosis should not be difficult, since the eye usually gives a fairly characteristic appearance. Headaches beginning in an older person previously free of headache always suggest the possibility of an organic explanation for the headache. This may be cranial arteritis or an organic intracranial process of some other nature.

SUMMARY

Headaches interfere with the quality of life of many people. Careful evaluation, with particular attention to a precise and detailed history, and appropriate medical and neurological examination will usually suffice to make the correct diagnosis. If the correct diagnosis is made, most patients can benefit from an appropriate management program. Physicians who are motivated to work with headache patients must be willing to commit the time needed to obtain the data necessary to make the diagnosis, and the time required to oversee a long-term management program. The clinician will find the results frequently quite rewarding.

14 Differential Diagnosis of Neck and Shoulder Pain

Jerome P. Reichmister

This chapter will address causes of neck and shoulder pain, including trauma and other conditions of the cervical spine which manifest as headache, neck pain, and shoulder and arm discomfort. As in any other medical problem the patient's history is of great importance. Bateman,[1] in his classic textbook on disorders of the shoulder and neck, categorized patients with pain as follows: 1) pain primarily in the neck, 2) neck-shoulder discomfort, 3) pain primarily in the shoulders, and 4) neck, shoulder, arm, hand and finger symptoms. Physical examination of the patient who presents with any of these complaints must include the neck, the root of the neck (which is the junction between the neck and the shoulder), the scapular and interscapular areas, pectoral regions, the clavicles, and the axilla.

Localized neck or suboccipital pain is mediated through the branches of the posterior primary rami of the spinal nerves and cervical plexus. The shoulder-neck pattern is also mediated through the posterior spinal nerve branches. The localized shoulder pain is mediated through the branches of the brachial plexus which go to the shoulder joint. The shoulder plus radiating pain symptoms (those that start in the neck and go distally into the arm and hand) are from nerve root or vascular irritation problems, and, therefore, are mediated through different pathways.

Discussion of localized neck disorders will include suboccipital arthritis, sternomastoid tendonitis, arthritis of the cervical spine, and chronic sprain. These four syndromes cause localized pain the the suboccipital and neck region. Viscerogenic causes will not be included in this discussion.

Suboccipital arthritis is usually due to degenerative changes which may occur in either the atlantoaxial or atlanto-occipital joints and usually occur secondary to trauma. The patient who has degenerative changes causing narrowing between the joints will present with pain to the area at the base of the skull. Characteristically, the patients with suboccipital arthritis have pain that really occurs early in movement of the head rather than in movement of the cervical spine. In the suboccipital region the pain is rather diffuse, and the slightest rotation, extension, or flexion may precipitate this discomfort. The discomfort begins with early motion before the lower cervical spine begins to move. Tenderness is usually felt in the suboccipital area and both sides of the midline rather than in the midline itself. It is frequently accompanied by a tendonitis of the erector spini muscles at their attachment in the suboccipital zone.

Some patients may have what is termed an "occipital neuralgia," which is mediated through the greater and lesser occipital nerves that pierce the musculature in the neck and distribute their end fibers into these areas. The pain of this type of neuralgia may radiate to the top of the head also.

Sternomastoid tendonitis is a derangement of the musculotendonous junction over the mastoid process. The patient has increased tone in the sternomastoid muscle. The pain is perceived behind the ear of the patient and is a rare condition. Characteristically, the pain is not related to rotation and the aching is more lateral than the discomfort noted in suboccipital arthritis. However, the tenderness is often unilateral and extends over the distal mastoid process. Occasionally, calcified streaking is reported in the muscles but it is rare.

Arthritis of the cervical spine is considered a normal development by middle age, but degenerative changes in the cervical spine may begin as early as age fifteen, according to DePalma et al.[2] It is important to note that if a patient has degenerative changes in the cervical spine by roentgenographic examination he may not be symptomatic. Chronic strain, injury, or debilitating disease may then trigger the pain in a patient with arthritis of the cervical spine. Other types of arthritis of the spine including rheumatoid arthritis may trigger symptoms in the cervico-occipital region. These patients may present with headaches. In patients with arthritic changes in the cervical spine, the pain is primarily due to neck motion and may extend into the shoulder. It is usually associated with stiffness and increases during the day. The patient frequently will show apprehension with turning the head and neck from side to side.

Patients with chronic sprain usually have had a whiplash injury, ie, an extension-flexion injury to the cervical spine. This diagnosis is criticized but is a real phenomenon. It is a result of probable tearing of the ligaments and muscle fibers in the cervical spine.

Occasionally, calcifications in the ligament near the tips of the spinous processes are seen. This is a different condition from the calcifications seen in the sternomastoid muscle. The patient may present with aching in the neck and discomfort across the shoulders. However, the discomfort is not related to shoulder motion, even though the complaint may be located mostly in the shoulder. The problem is mainly in the lower neck and is episodic in nature. The tenderness is localized in the ligamentous area and is directly related to the spinous processes. At times, these patients will complain of a crackling sensation in the neck when they turn their head and neck.

The neck-shoulder pattern is pain in the neck-shoulder location, and is usually described as aching and gnawing in character. It is usually difficult for these patients to localize their discomfort, except that they may enter the office holding the neck-shoulder area and complaining that this is the region that is uncomfortable for them. This pain is sometimes described as sharp and grabbing and it even may produce some tingling. It may be associated with postural disturbances, fibrositis, scapulothoracic disorders, and neurologic disturbances. The postural disturbances result from strain on the muscles that are required to keep the head erect and to support the upper extremities. Poor posture, round shoulders, and pendulous breasts may be associated with this phenomenon; often, patients have bilateral complaints.

The fibrositis or myofascial syndrome is a collection of musculotendonous disorders which usually are chronic. These may develop sequelae in either occupational or habitual shoulder strains or may even occur secondary to trauma. These patients may exhibit nodular thickening in the trapezius muscles and other muscles in the region such as the levator scapulae, the rhomboids, and in the erector spini. These nodular areas are often very tender. It is possible that these patients may have occipital headache associated with this phenomenon. This is no acute distress associated with neck or shoulder motion in these patients, but they do have localized trigger zones which may be relieved by injection into the trigger points. The best way to examine a patient with localized nodular thickening and suspected fibrositis or myofascial syndrome is when the patient is prone and relaxed.

Neurological disturbances are mentioned here so that they will be kept in mind. One must look for shoulder girdle weakness, shoulder girdle atrophy, and a feeling of heaviness in the neck and shoulder areas. Other neurologic disturbances such as accessory nerve paralysis, deltoid paralysis, and progressive muscular atrophy must also be borne in mind.

The shoulder plus radiating pain pattern includes several problem areas. This discussion will be limited to the cervical root syndrome as others present more with shoulder, arm, and hand complaints. Cervical root syndrome is caused by extruded and degenerative discs as well as foraminal compression and spondylotic changes. Cord tumor and fractures form a very small percentage of root syndrome problems. The pain originates in the neck and then progresses distally. The patients complain of sharp, shooting pains which are aggravated by coughing, sneezing, and neck motion. The pain pattern is usually fairly specific along dermatomal patterns; for example, the C-5 neurological level is associated with a disc problem between C-4 and C-5. An excellent reference on this subject is a concise book written for orthopedists, Hoppenfeld.[3] The key differential point to be considered when root problems are present is the difference between the pain of this phenomenon and the pain and symptoms from a cervical cord tumor. Tumors will have a gradual onset of pain and will be unrelieved by the classic modalities of rest and other conservative measures. There may be increased tone in the lower extremities with tumors and a positive Babinski sign and clonus. Cerebral spinal fluid analysis shows increased protein levels with tumors. Other diagnostic tests such as electromyography (EMG), nerve conduction studies, and myelography are helpful.

Disc pain is not as severe and usually not as intractable as the pain seen with tumor. There is local pain in the neck plus radiating pain to the arm. Often these patients have intermittent bouts of discomfort that are relieved with rest, by the use of a cervical collar, hot packs, massage, trigger point injections, analgesics, anti-inflammatory medications, muscle relaxants and other conservative modalities. Motion increases the pain in the patient who has disc problems. Tilting the head toward the side of the disc lesion will increase the pain; however, tilting the head away from the side of the disc lesion usually will decrease the pain. Characteristic root patterns and reflex, motor, and sensory changes are seen. In these patients, the workup should include EMG, nerve conduction studies, neurosurgical consultation, and myelography. Thermography is sometimes helpful also.

Foraminal encroachment is seen in the older age group and is usually secondary to chronic degenerative disc disease. These patients first complain of neck and shoulder discomfort and then of radiating pain down the arms. This neck discomfort also manifests as suboccipital headache. Sometimes, these patient's symptoms are not obvious and they will lack clear-cut motor and sensory deficits. Obviously, x-ray films are very helpful, particularly the oblique x-ray studies which show the foraminal encroachment. Electromyography, nerve conduction studies, and myelography should also be included in the evaluation of patients with this disorder.

An interesting follow-up study of 6000 cases of chronic headache was reported in 1975 by Braaf and Rosner.[4] The follow-up was carried out from 2 to 25 years after the cessation of treatment. There is a sexual predominance; women seem to have more problems with chronic headache than do males. The age of the group ranged from 8 to 70 years. The duration of the headaches was between 1 and 56 years, the average duration being 15 years. It is interesting to note that the authors discuss cervical trauma as a cause of chronic headache. In a review of the literature in 1942, Kelly[5] was the first to mention that chronic cervical problems were a cause of headache. Raney and Raney,[6] in 1948, noted that many of those patients operated upon for cervical disc lesions who had positive myelograms also complained of headaches. Goff et al[7] and Gay and Abbot[8] also stressed injury to the neck as the cause of chronic headache and included several factors in their study: trauma, heredity, allergy, and a large group of miscellaneous factors. Forty-four percent of the 6000 patients had a positive history of trauma to the neck. Some were caused by direct trauma to the neck; others were caused by indirect trauma including whiplash, a fall on the outstretched hand, or a fall down the steps. Often, the patients do not remember this trauma; thus, it is important to take a careful medical history. The patient may not associate the trauma with his headache because the onset of the headache may be delayed for weeks, or even months. From the literature it is not completely understood what role heredity plays in headache. However, 30% of the 6000 patients gave a positive family history of headaches. Interestingly, however, in 40% of these cases there was antecedent neck trauma. Allergy has often been considered an etiologic factor in headache because of the frequent association of certain drugs and foods with headache. Thirty-three percent of the patients studied had an allergy to a particular food. However, this allergy developed after the traumatic incident, which usually was whiplash.

The miscellaneous group includes menopause, emotional disturbances, tension, constipation, drugs, alcohol, and cold drafts. Prolonged writing or reading, vacuuming, and lifting and carrying were also cited as causes of chronic headache usually seen by orthopedic surgeons. A possible explanation for these problems has been thought to have been related to indirect strain in the cervical trapezius areas. The physical findings include localized tenderness, varying degrees of spasm, and a reduced range of motion. Digital pressure may initiate or aggravate an attack in this type of patient.

Braaf and Rosner[4] also studied x-ray films. They believed that the loss of the lordotic curve of the cervical region was very important, as well as the narrowing of the disc spaces, hypertrophic lipping of contiguous vertebral bodies, and changes in the vertebral foramen. Loss of the lordotic curve is questionable. It is true that some people have a loss of the cervical lordotic curve secondary to injury or muscle spasm, but it is also possible to see loss of the cervical lordotic curve on an x-ray film simply by positioning the head and neck in various manners. Therefore, it seems that their emphasis on the loss of the cervical lordotic curve is somewhat a moot point. In treating headaches, the orthopedist first eliminates other causes of headaches, then considers the cervical area as a possible source.

If conservative outpatient treatment has failed to relieve headache which is thought to be cervical in origin, the patient may be offered admission to the hospital for 7 to 10 days of continuous traction, and then have intermittent cervical traction as an outpatient. In treating patients with cervical problems, the most useful drugs are aspirin and other mild analgesics and muscle relaxants. The cervical collar, heat, massage, and neck strengthening exercises are also effective treatments. In the patient with intractable headache thought to be of cervical origin, and in whom all avenues of outpatient diagnosis and therapy have been exhausted, one must consider a myelogram, discometry, or possibly even surgery.

Braaf and Rosner[4] reviewed 15 articles on neck discomfort and headaches and found that patients who have had headache for less than one year in duration responded very well to cervical traction, with 90% reporting excellent relief. Of those patients with headaches for one to five years, 80% experienced excellent relief with traction, 15% reported some improvement, and 5% received no benefit at all from the cervical traction. In patients with headache for 5 to 56 years, improvement was noted in 60% with the use of cervical traction.

Headache as a referred symptom of cervical origin may be caused by prior injury to the neck. It is the opinion of the author that this type of headache is extremely important to discuss. The headache may be also caused by degenerative disease of the cervical spine. The structures that are affected are muscles, fascia, ligaments, discs, nerve roots, vertebral vessels, and the cervical sympathetic chain. When a disc is injured, there is a narrowing of the disc space and subsequent narrowing of the facet joints. Hypertrophic spurring of the contiguous vertebral bodies occurs, followed by encroachment of the vertebral foramen. The patient may suffer from irritation of the cervical roots, vertebral vessels, and sympathetic plexus.

Discs can be injured as a result of chronic ligamentous stretch and strain. The upper cervical spinal nerves are intimately connected to the last three cranial nerves through the autonomic nervous system. Patients often complain of bizarre visceral symptoms, such as nausea, vertigo, or symptoms compatible with compression of the vertebral arteries. The problem on an intermittent basis may cause partial ischemia and disturbance of the circulation to the occipital lobe of the cerebral cortex and the cerebellum and even give rise to symptoms of cranial nerve dysfunction. Braaf and Rosner[4] believe that the sympathetic nerves are affected either directly by torsion or even indirectly by reflex action. Mechanical derangement of the cervical spine may irritate or stimulate the cervical roots, the cervical cranial autonomic nervous system, and the vertebral vessels all of which can cause headaches and a wide range of other symptoms.

One may wonder about surgical experience with cervical discogenic headache. Surgery is not the treatment of choice for all cervical discogenic headache. When the cervical headache is associated with other symptoms of cervical disc disease, the results are much better than the surgical experience for patients who present only the symptoms of cervical headache. To clarify this point, when a patient is operated upon for headache alone believed to be due to a cervical cause the results at best are equivocal. If the patient has headache and radicular symptoms and signs in the upper extremities, the results will be better. In describing the mechanism of relief for cervical discogenic headaches, it is the author's belief that there is a definitive surgical procedure. This consists of removal of the disc and replacing it with a bone graft, achieving a solid fusion and distracting the vertebral bodies. Opening up the vertebral foramen will bring about a relaxation of the spastic muscles in the cervical spine, thereby splinting the diseased cervical spine. Again, it is stressed that the best results are obtained in those patients who have not only cervical discogenic headache but symptoms of cervical radiculopathy in the upper extremities.

It is important to stress the necessity of obtaining and recording a complete and careful history. Psychogenic factors and intracranial problems must be ruled out before surgery. Obviously, histamine and vascular tension states and other causes presented in Chapter 13 are important to consider when dealing with this problem. It is wise to use cervical traction before surgery is considered and also to use a trial of a cervical two-poster brace as a form of immobilization to ascertain relief of the headache symptoms.

REFERENCES

1. Bateman JE: *The Shoulder and Neck.* Philadelphia, WB Saunders Co, 1972.
2. DePalma AF, Rothman RH: *The Intervertebral Disc.* Philadelphia, WB Saunders Co, 1970.
3. Hoppenfeld S: *Orthopaedic Neurology—A Diagnostic Guide to Neurologic Levels.* Philadelphia, JB Lippincott, 1977.
4. Braaf M, Rosner S: Trauma of cervical spine as cause of chronic headaches. *J Trauma* 1975;15:441–445.

5. Kelly M: Headaches, traumatic and rheumatic:The cervical somatic lesion. *Med J Aust* 1942;2:479.
6. Raney AA, Raney RB: Headaches:A common symptom of cervical disc lesions. *Arch Neurol Psych* 1945;59:603–621.
7. Goff CW, Aldes JH, Alden IO: *Traumatic Cervical Syndrome and Whiplash.* Philadelphia, JB Lippincott, 1964, p 22.
8. Gay JR, Abbott KH: Common whiplash injuries of the neck. *JAMA* 1953;152:1698.

15 Myofacial Pain Dysfunction Syndrome

Jerome D. Buxbaum

The purpose of this chapter is to give the reader a reasonable overview of those orofacial structures involved in myofacial pain (MPD) syndrome. The author's goal is to provide sufficient information to aid in making a differential diagnosis. There is no attempt to provide treatment modes. That should properly be done by a clinician specializing in the field.

Myofacial pain syndrome was first recognized in 1934, when Costens, an otolaryngologist, astutely recognized a family of symptoms including pain which affected orofacial structures. It was originally termed "Costens syndrome." As more information was amassed the name changed first to temporomandibular joint syndrome, and then finally to myo-orofacial pain syndrome, or, more popularly, myofacial pain dysfunction syndrome (MPD).

The prevalence of this pathologic entity is extremely high and widespread. Epidemiologic studies in a number of countries are remarkably similar and show that between 50% to 60% of the populations studied demonstrated some MPD symptomatology.[1] Although any age group may be involved, women between 20 to 50 years of age comprise the largest group seeking treatment. It has been postulated that differences in the general adaptive syndrome between men and women may account for the disparity.

As will be shown later, these individuals present with a variety of symptoms. Their histories are often complex and involved. Frequently they will report previous treatment by physician, otolaryngologist, neurologist, neurosurgeon, psychiatrist, and dentist. Sometimes, they make the cycle more than once.

In order to evaluate the possibility of MPD syndrome and make a meaningful referral, it is necessary to understand the physiologic composition of the involved structures.

Components of the System

It is essential to know that the stomatognathic system is a closed interrelated system consisting of four parts. These parts are the temporomandibular joint (TMJ), the dentition, the periodontium, and the associated neuromusculature. These four parts must function within the physiologic tolerances of the patient in order for orofacial health to be maintained. In addition, it is also important to realize that any change in one component will cause immediate changes in one or more of the other components in the system. These changes may or may not be of a magnitude to produce clinical symptomatology. However, it is important to explore this interdependence in the examination. The examiner should determine whether the patient had any dental treatment or orthodontia prior to the onset of symptoms and establish their temporal relationship with symptoms. The patient should also be questioned about any exposure to general anesthesia since intubation can markedly affect the system.

The Temporomandibular Joint And Its Relation to Otic Structure

In phylogenetic development, the jaw joint developed its modifications in response to evolutionary changes in locomotion and dietary composition. The most primitive vertebrate jaw consists of a simple hinge derived from the first visceral arch. This joint form allowed very limited motion, simple open and close. As the demand for mobility increased the dentate bone went through an entire phylogenetic pattern of change. One important step in this process was the penetration of skull to form a joint, superior in relation to the dentition. This joint consisted of newer and fewer structures. The dentate bone became smaller and smaller and starting with the amphibian became part of the otic structure.

In man, the hyomandibular bone became the stapes, the quadrate bone and incus, and the articulare bone, the malleus.[2(p6)] In essence then, what the dentate bone was prehistorically became the osseous structures of the ear in man. This intimate relation between the TMJ and otic structures is based on evolutionary fact. The tensor tympani muscle which moves the malleus is a vestige of the muscle which once moved the jaw. It is innervated by a branch of the motor division of cranial nerve V (trigeminal nerve). In addition, the malleomandibular ligament (Pinto's ligament) connects the neck and anterior process of the malleus to the temporomandibular joint capsule and miniscus. Burch[3] has shown that this ligament is a continuation of the sphenomandibular ligament of the temporomandibular joint.

The eustachian tube also is related anatomically to the TMJ. Superiorly, the tube lies in close approximation to the tensor tympani muscle. Through most of its length the walls of the tube are in contact. They are opened during the act of swallowing primarily by the tensor veli palatini muscle. This muscle is innervated by a branch of the motor division of cranial nerve V. The joint itself lies in close approximation to most otic structures.

Thus, the otic symptomatology such as tinnitus, stuffiness, pain, and vertigo have a multiple anatomic and physiologic basis from pathology in the stomatognathic system. This statement must be taken in context. Certainly, many pathologic conditions may produce otic symptomatology. Entire texts have been written on vertigo and its diagnostic possibilities, including psychologic, which this symptom suggests. However, if otic symptoms are present and no otic pathology is discernible, then MPD syndrome must be considered a viable diagnostic possibility.

General Description of the TMJ

The temporomandibular joint is classified as a ginglymoarthrodial joint. That is, the joint is capable of both translation and rotation. At present, there is some question as to whether or not there is any pure rotary movement of the joint. However this question is not relevant to the objectives of this text.

The joint is synovial. It consists of the head of the condyle of the mandible, and a biconcave miniscus or articular disc which articulates with the articular eminence of the temporal bone (see Figure 15-1). This line of articulation is physiologically harmonious with the trabecular pattern in both the condylar head and articular eminence as well as the force vectors in the mandibular elevator muscles.

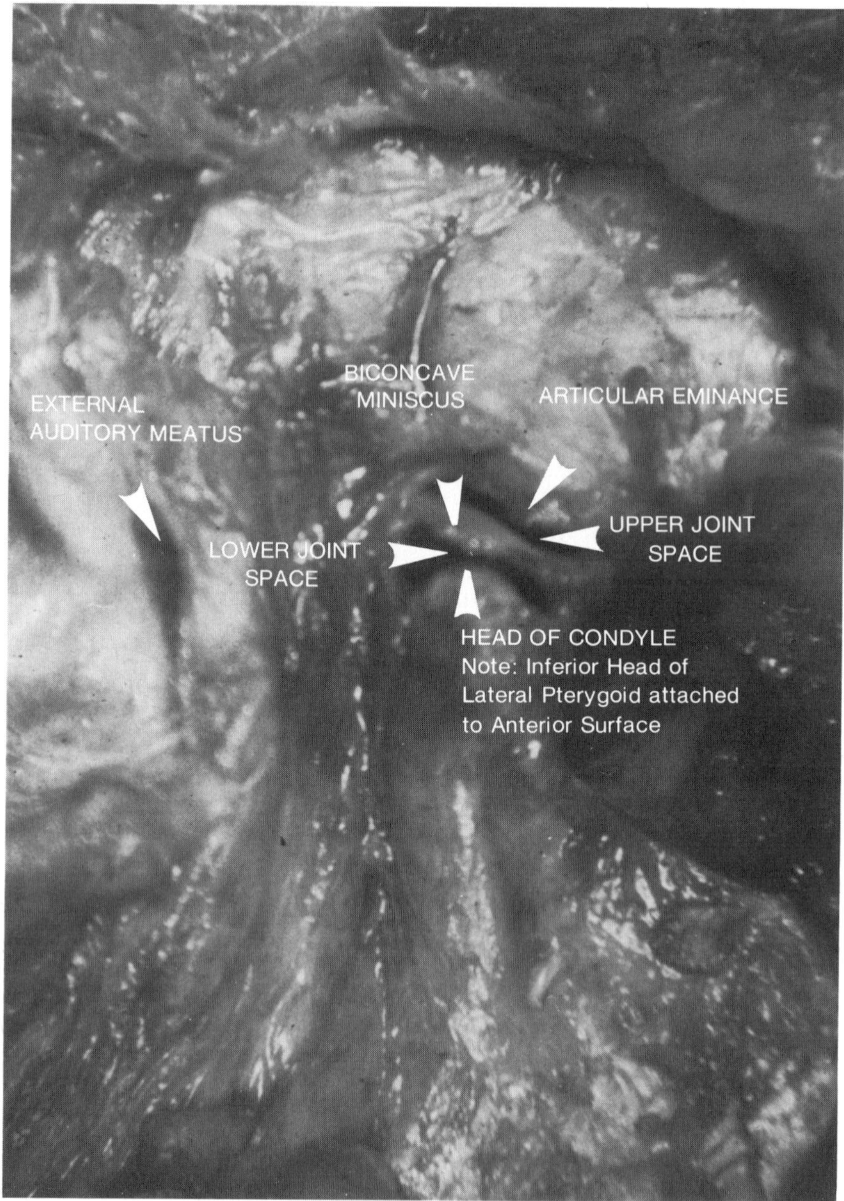

Figure 15-1 Articulator components of the temporomandibular joint.

In the younger healthy joint the miniscus is rather snugly attached to the medial and lateral aspects of the condylar head. Because of this attachment to the head of the condyle, the miniscus translates with it as the condylar head translates down the articular eminence. Jaw opening is initiated by the inferior head of the lateral pterygoid. Downward and forward movement of the miniscus produces an unfolding of the synovial membrane and a stretching of the elastin fibers of the bilaminar zone. During closure of the mandible, the superior head of the lateral pterygoid becomes active. Its contraction counter balances the pull of the elastin fibers. Thus, it always keeps the thin central portion of the miniscus interposed between the condylar head and the articular eminence.[4]

In the compromised state the miniscus is no longer in tight approximation with the head of the condyle. This condition may be the result of an acute traumatic experience such as an accident or an extraction. These traumas tend to drive the condylar head posteriorly and superiorly, thereby stretching the attachment and loosening the disc. In addition, chronic stress on the joint due primarily to disharmonies in the occlusal interface will produce over long periods of time, the same looseness in the disc attachment.

The presence of a loosely attached disc forms the basis for the clicking symptoms that effect so many MPD patients. There are several theories as to the cause of clicking, but their presentation is beyond the scope of our discussion. In essence, the click represents the condylar head slipping over the rim of the miniscus. Clicking is demonstrable evidence of muscle incoordination.[2]

Uniqueness of the Temporomandibular Joint

The temporomandibular joint is unique in five different ways:

1. The articular surfaces are covered with fibrocartilage. Fibrocartilage is usually associated with joints which have limited movement.
2. It is the only heavy weight-bearing joint which permits such a wide and diverse range of rotary and translatory movements.
3. It is an extremely mobile bilateral articulation. It is not two separate and distinct joints because the mandible is a solid body. There can be no movement in one temporomandibular joint which does not result in some compensatory movement in the contralateral joint. It is in reality one joint with two articulations.
4. The osseous structures contain teeth. The intercuspal position of the dentition stops closure. All other joints have

only ligaments which stop closure. If the dentition prevents the elevator musculature from achieving 57% of its resting length, then isotonic contraction is converted to isometric contraction. This is not a desired condition. Of equal importance is the fact that the dentition with its sensory receptors programs the closing pathway of the mandible by its influence on the neuromusculature. For a healthy state to exist the dentition must not interfere with the physiologic operation of the neuromusculature.

5. It is the only joint which displays fulcal transference. When a bolus or other object is placed between the maxillary and mandibular dentition and closure force is exerted, the fulcrum of the lever action of the joint shifts.

Sensory Receptors of the Temporomandibular Joint

Wyke[5] has identified four distinct receptor types that are found within the capsule of the temporomandibular joint. Type I receptors are responsive to both static and dynamic states. They are low threshold, slowly adapting receptors. Type II receptors are dynamic low threshold, rapidly adapting mechanoreceptors. Type III receptors are high threshold, slowly adapting mechanoreceptors. Type IV receptors are high threshold, nonadapting pain receptors.

The result of this rich mechanoreceptor representation is that the joint capsule itself is capable of and, in fact, routinely does influence the neuromuscular response of the skeletal muscles associated with it. The joint is not merely a passive responder to muscle activity but to an important degree determines the muscular activity.

Some Clinical Effects of TMJ Physiology

The stress bearing aspects of the joint are relatively avascular and have a meager neural supply. Therefore, notable joint pathology can occur without producing marked symptomatology. The poor vascular supply means that repair and healing in the stress bearing areas is a slow process. Any form of therapy which produces a dramatic rapid remission of symptoms means that the symptom causing pathology could not exist in the essential joint structures.

In the medial portion of the anterior section of the capsule, the only support is provided by loose areolar connective tissue. Therefore, traumatic whiplash injuries easily result in hypertranslation of the condyles, with associated injury to other soft tissue structures.

Similar damage is produced on intubation. Muscle relaxant drugs are administered to ease the intubation process, but without care on the part of the anesthesiologist extensive damage may be done to the structures of the stomatognathic system.

Musculature Associated With Mandibular Movement

The muscles associated with mandibular movement may be divided into four groups for purposes of discussion. However, in function these groups operate as a well-integrated continuum.

What is commonly called the masticatory musculature includes the superficial and deep masseter, anterior, middle and posterior temporali, internal (medial) pterygoid, and external (lateral) pterygoid. With the exception of the lateral pterygoid, all of the other masticatory muscles are primarily mandibular elevators.

The lateral pterygoid is involved with initiating mandibular opening as well as controlling all lateral and lateral protrusive movements. The muscle consists of a small superior head which inserts on the miniscus, or articular disc, and a larger inferior head which inserts on the anterior portion of the neck of the condyle.

The anatomic arrangement just described provides the clinician with the opportunity to make some revealing observations. Ask the patient to close the teeth together normally. Then, look to see if the midlines of the maxillary and mandibular dentition are in line with one another. Although midline deviation may be the result of tooth position, it may also be the result of spasm in the lateral pterygoids. In either event, the patient should be referred to a specialist to determine the etiology of midline deviation.

Ask the patient to open the mouth slowly. Does the mandible deviate from a straight downward movement? Deviation to one side is usually caused by spasm in the contralateral lateral pterygoid. This condition also requires referral for diagnosis and treatment.

Clicks are often the result of neuromuscular incoordination. If a patient presents with an audible click associated with mandibular deviation, a simple exercise can often provide relief. If the maxillary and mandibular midlines are in alignment, place a stimudent between the maxillary central incisors and another stimudent between the mandibular central incisors. Give the patient a mirror and have him open and close the mandible, keeping the stimudents in line. If the click is of uncomplicated neuromuscular origin, it will disappear. These muscles are all innervated by branches of the motor division of cranial nerve V (the trigeminal). Although mandibular opening is initiated by the lateral (external) pterygoids, it is completed by the supra- and infrahyoid muscle groups.

The suprahyoid group consists of the digastric (anterior and posterior belly), mylohyoid, geniohyoid, and stylohyoid muscles. The major function of these muscles as a group is to depress the mandible. However, as their origin is mainly the hyoid bone, this bone must be fixed or stabilized by the infrahyoid musculature. The innervation of the suprahyoid group is varied. The posterior belly of the digastric is supplied by cranial nerve VII (facial nerve) and the anterior belly by a branch of the motor division of cranial nerve V. The mylohyoid is also supplied by the fifth cranial nerve. The geniohyoid is innervated by cranial nerve XII (hypoglossal), and the stylohyoid by the facial nerve VII.

It was noted above that the hyoid bone must be stabilized by the infrahyoid muscles to allow the suprahyoids to fulfill their action. The infrahyoid muscles consist of the omohyoid, sternohyoid, sternothyroid, and thyrohyoid. The thyrohyoid is innervated by the hypoglossal nerve. The remaining infrahyoids are innervated by cervical nerves 1 to 3 (the ansa hypoglossi).

The associated musculature plays an interactive role in the response to the actions of the muscle groups already described. Davies[6] and others have conclusively demonstrated that the sternocleidomastoid, trapezius, and semispinalis capitus muscles play an essential role in mandibular movement. If the head is tilted upward as in looking at the sky, the mandible is depressed. If we turn our heads to one side, the mandible deviates contralaterally. There can be no question that myositic activity in one of these muscle groups has a ripple effect, producing alterations in the activity of all the muscles involved in mandibular movement. This ripple effect covers other muscles innervated by cranial nerve V, such as the tensor tympani and tensor villi pallatini. The platysma is another muscle associated with mandibular movement, as one of its prime actions is to aid in mandibular depression.

To illustrate the complexity of the system, the simple act of depressing the mandible involves a minimum of 18 pairs of muscles and six major nerve trunks, all acting in a smoothly coordinated fashion (see Figure 15-2).

The Genesis of Myospasm

There are over 100 different pathologic entities which can produce MPD symptomatology. Of these, myositis or muscle spasm is one of the most important. Some authorities believe 70% to 80% of patients

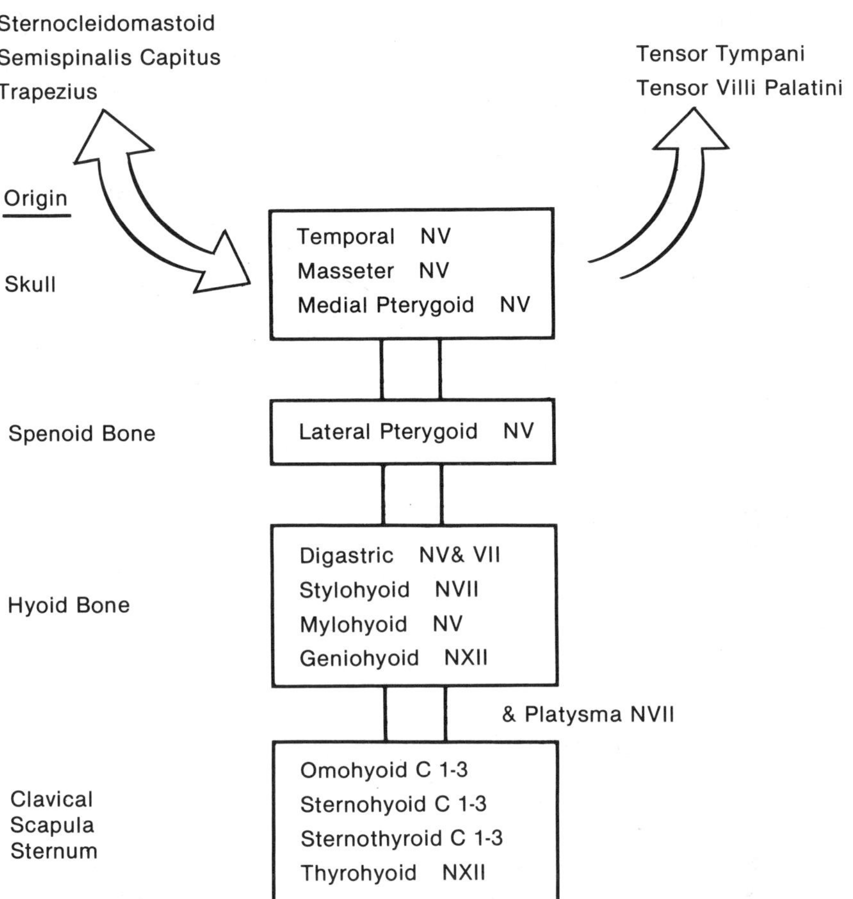

Figure 15-2 A diagram of the major muscles involved with mandibular movement.

presenting with MPD problems fall into the myositic category.[7]

In order to understand muscle spasm, some of the basic principles of skeletal muscle physiology must be reviewed. The author does not intend to present a total view of the anatomy and physiology of skeletal muscle activity. The reader is referred to Guyton's text.[8]

Ample amounts of adenosinetriphosphate (ATP) must be present in the skeletal muscle fiber in order for *both* actin-myosin binding (the contractile process) and decoupling (the relaxation process) to take place. ATP is present in the cytoplasm and nucleoplasm of almost every cell. This enzyme is derived from foodstuffs by means of a series of complex biochemical reactions. It can be used and reused countless times.

Although all foodstuffs can be used to produce ATP, the greatest and most efficient supply is obtained from carbohydrate metabolism under aerobic conditions. To illustrate this point aerobically, 1 mole of glucose (180 g) will yield 686,000 calories. Under anaerobic conditions the same mole of glucose yields only 16,000 calories. Only 8000 calories are required to produce 1 g mole of ATP. Therefore, it would be totally inefficient if glucose were decomposed in one step to water and CO_2 while forming a single ATP molecule. The body avoids this by having the decomposition take place gradually through the processes of glycolysis with the formation of pyruvic acid, the conversion of pyruvic acid to acetyl coenzyme A, the Krebs cycle, and oxidative phosphorylization. The result of these degradation processes is that each mole of glucose produces 38 moles of ATP.[9]

Under nominal conditions the mechanism just described produces normal contraction and relaxation of skeletal muscle fibers. The efferent (motor) nerve depolarizes. The action potential is transmitted to the skeletal muscle fiber by means of the myoneural junction, and the muscle fibers respond.

However, under prolonged or abnormal contraction, two events occur which disrupt the normal pattern. These two events are ATP depletion and vasoconstriction. The ATP supply can be depleted within seconds. The contractile process reduces the diameter of the associated vascular bed and thus produces a vasoconstrictive situation. These two phenomena produce almost complete muscle fatigue within one minute. The neural supply still remains operative. The myoneural junction is still capable of normal transmission, but the muscle response becomes more diminished due to disruption of its normal metabolic process.

Diagramatically, the genesis of myospasm is depicted in Figure 15-3. There are six known factors which tend to influence the onset of myospasm and include:

- Nutritional
- Noxious stimulation
- Mechanical
- Emotional
- Infectious
- Metabolic

A localized area of spastic skeletal muscle fibers is called a trigger zone. By definition, the trigger zone is a small hypersensitive area, from which afferent impulses bombard the central nervous system and give rise to an area of referred pain. We have a predictable anatomic pathway of pain symptoms, manifested at some distance from the associated trigger zone. The referred pain areas for the head and neck have been meticulously mapped out by Travell,[10] and we are indebted to the contribution she has made to our understanding of these phenomena.

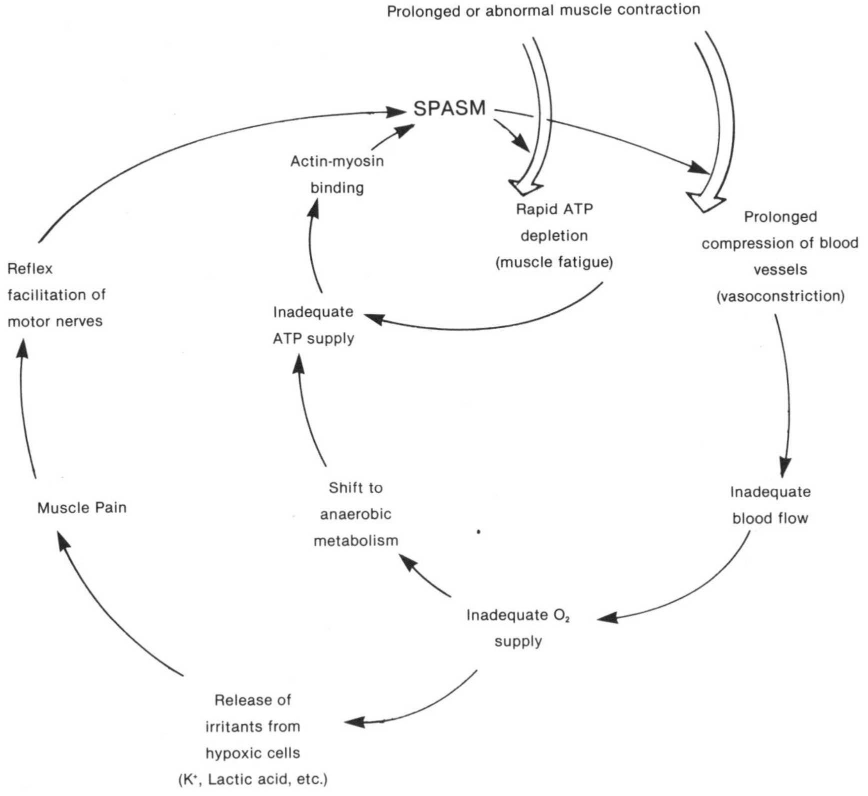

Figure 15-3 The myospastic cycle.

One probable sequence of events producing myospasm in the masticatory system would be as follows. The patient attempts to close the mandible into a functional position that is physiologically acceptable to the neuromusculature. The occlusal interface (that is, the anatomy of the occluding surfaces of the maxillary and mandibular dentition) interposes an interference to this ideal pathway. When the interference point (prematurity) is reached in the closure path, excessive pressure is transmitted through the tooth and is detected by mechanoreceptors and pain receptors in the periodontal ligament. These mechanoreceptors via central nervous system connections, which will be described later in the chapter, alter the closure pathway to protect the tooth with the prematurity from injury. The proprioceptive change in closure pattern may also come, as previously noted, from receptors located in the joint capsule itself. The mandible assumes a convenience position which may be beyond the physiologically acceptable limits of the neuromusculature.

The ligaments and joint capsule are also affected. The affected structures constantly attempt to return to a normal pattern but end up in a conflict with the dentition. The end result of this conflict is often incoordinated muscle activity, abnormal function, and muscle spasm. The formation of the initial area of myospasm comprises just one part of a more involved pain phenomena. As noted before, the myospastic areas become trigger points which give rise to areas of referred pain. The referred pain site may persist even after the stimulus and initial area of spasm have been corrected. In fact, the referred pain site may produce myospastic activity in other areas.

Clinical Notes on Myospasm

There are several important factors to be considered when applying the physiology of myospasm to the clinical examination. The neuromuscular system develops muscle memory. This is the result of synaptic characteristics and we see its obvious application in the golf swing or tennis stroke. The same pattern program applies to mandibular closure pathways. Therefore, simply asking the patient to close the teeth together will reveal only the habitual closure pattern. Specialized techniques are necessary to determine if any occlusal disharmony exists.

Muscle palpation can be mastered by any clinician. There are several excellent audiovisual teaching tapes in this area.[11] One vital fact to remember is that when palpating the masticatory and associated musculature the mouth should be kept in an open position. This can easily be achieved by inserting a rubber stopper of appropriate size between the anterior teeth.

Receptors

Think for a moment about the amount and range of body control that is necessary when we walk over uneven terrain like the sand dunes on a beach. In order to control this type of movement, the central nervous system (CNS) receives input information from several sources. The optic system supplies visual information. The vestibular apparatus helps maintain balance. However, in order for the system to function, there must be a rapid and continuous flow of information regarding tension and length from the muscles themselves. This flow of information is termed feedback. Feedback provides for rapid adjustment of the control system in accordance with the changing lengths and tensions of muscles.

It has been estimated that during mastication over 100,000 signals per sec are generated by the feedback receptors. Four different receptors have been identified which are involved in the feedback process. These are muscle spindles, Golgi tendon organs, free nerve endings, and pachinian corpuscles. The receptors in the joint capsule have been classified by Wyke,[5] as noted previously. However, Types I, II, and III may be considered analagous to the other mechanoreceptors just listed. Although an indepth discussion of receptors is not germane to this presentation, two of the receptors should be briefly described. The reader is urged to read further about this important topic.[12(p227)]

The muscle spindle consists of about six rudimentary skeletal muscle fibers. These fibers are called intrafusal fibers. The spindle lies in parallel with the extrafusal skeletal muscle fibers. The spindle has a dual sensory innervation consisting of a primary afferent (A-alpha) and a secondary (A-beta) nerve fiber. As the muscle is stretched, the spindle is stretched and this change is transmitted by the sensory nerves just described into the central nervous system. There, the sensory neuron makes a synaptic connection with an alpha motor neuron. The alpha motor neuron then returns to the skeletal muscle fiber and contraction occurs. This is a simplistic description of the myotatic or stretch reflex. To recapitulate, the sequence of events is:

1. Stretch of the muscle fibers which causes the spindles to be stretched.
2. The stretch activates the sensory neurons attached to the spindle.
3. The sensory neuron enters the central nervous system and makes a synaptic connection with an alpha motor neuron.
4. The alpha motor neuron returns to the muscle and triggers its contraction.

In addition to two sensory innervations, the spindle also receives two efferent nerves. These are called gamma S and gamma D efferents and are located at either end of the spindle (see Figure 15-4). Their effect is called gamma loop or gamma biasing. When the gamma efferents are activated, they stretch the intrafusal fibers of the spindle without the muscle itself being stretched. Their effect is extremely important. They affect load and damping reflexes,[6] and literally fine tune the muscle response. Because of the gamma loop system, exercise regimes for MPD patients should be gently and slowly performed.

The Golgi tendon organ (GTO) is arranged in series with the extrafusal muscle fibers. It is usually found between the muscle fibers and the tendon. The GTO is responsive to active tension and is, therefore, an inhibitory type of receptor concerned primarily with protection of the muscle.

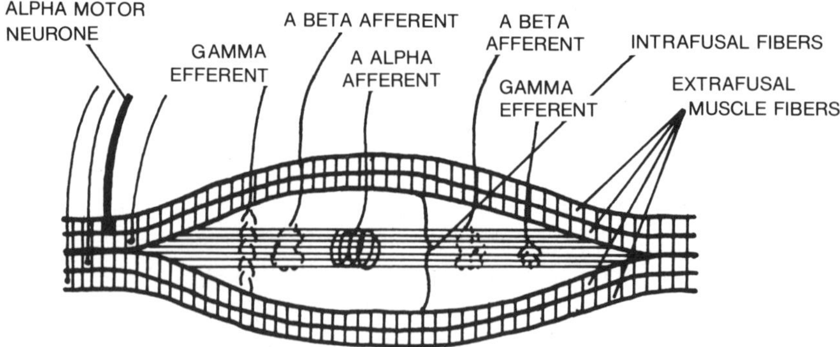

Figure 15-4 Diagram of a muscle spindle receptor.

Overview of the Neurophysiology of the Trigeminal Nerve

For an indepth description of cranial nerve V, the reader is referred to Dubner et al.[12] The locus of almost all first order neuron cell bodies of the trigeminal nerve is the semilunar or gasserian ganglion. From this ganglion the three peripheral projections are the ophthalmic, maxillary, and mandibular divisions of the trigeminal nerve.

The central projections from the first order neurons enter the central nervous system and make synaptic connections with second order neurons in either the chief (main sensory) nucleus or the spinal nucleus. The spinal nucleus has been divided cytoarchitecturally into three subnuclei. The most rostral is the subnucleus oralis followed by the subnucleus interpolaris; the most caudally located one is the subnucleus caudalis.

Nerve fibers associated with the transmission of pain descend after leaving the semilunar ganglion and make their synaptic connections primarily in subnucleus caudalis. (Some pain fibers do make synaptic connections in interpolaris and oralis.) In addition to synaptic relays for cranial nerve V in the nucleus caudalis, the same nucleus also has synaptic relays for facial nerve (VII), hypoglossal nerve (XII), vagus nerve (X), and cervical nerves 1 to 3. This neuronal arrangement could provide a basis for some of the observed referred pain pathways.

Other Nuclei Involved with Trigeminal Nerve Activity

Mechanoreceptive sensations from the periodontal ligaments and portions of the gingiva pass over heavily myelinated nerve fibers directly through the semilunar ganglion to their first order neurons, which are located in the mesencephalic nucleus of the trigeminal nerve. This is perhaps the only location of first order neurons within the central nervous system. The synapses within the nucleus are also unique. Almost all other synapses in the nervous system are neuronal in character. That is, both the pre- and postsynaptic units maintain an intact cell membrane. Transmission is accomplished by chemical mediators (either excitatory or inhibitory) across a synaptic cleft. In the mesencephalic nucleus the synapses are gap-junction. This means some protoplasmic continuity between pre- and postsynaptic units with an associated reduction in transmission delay. Postsynaptic projections from the mesencephalic nucleus either make monosynaptic connections with the motor nucleus of the trigeminal nerve or ascend to higher thalamic and cortical levels.

What has just been described is a rapidly conducting, high fidelity pathway from the mechanoreceptors of dental and oral structures to the mesencephalic nucleus and to the motor nucleus, producing an efferent response in the jaw closing musculature. It is the pathway over which the closure patterns previously described are generated.

In addition to the mesencephalic and motor nucleus, the trigeminal complex also contains the supratrigeminal nucleus. This nucleus is primarily involved with inhibitory types of muscle response.

The Modality of Pain as Applied to Dental and Facial Structures

Dental and facial pain can be divided into three distinct components. Based on effect, these components are: 1) actual perception of the pain, 2) motor responses to the pain, and 3) the cortical interpretation of the pain.[13(p25)] These three components are represented by three separate neuroanatomic pathways which start from the subnucleus caudalis.

Pain can also be divided on the basis of origin. Under this division the sources are the peripheral area, the brainstem, and the corticothalamic region. It is most important to remember that regardless of the origin of the pain any or all of the components can be manifested in the patient. In addition, all of the psychopathologic entities which are about to be categorized fall under the broad umbrella term of myofacial pain dysfunction syndrome.

Pain of peripheral origin This type of pain is divided into four categories, musculoskeletal, vascular, dental-facial, and neural.

The musculoskeletal division includes pain from:

1. Fractures
2. Trauma
3. Rheumatoid arthritis of the TMJ

4. Osteoarthritis of the TMJ
5. Degeneration of the miniscus (disc)
6. Skeletal anomalies
7. Tumors
8. Infectious (osseous cavitation)[14]
9. Myospasm
10. Primary trigger points and referred pain
11. Secondary trigger points and referred pain

Muscular pain is the most common and accounts for pain in from 60% to 80% of patients.

Pain from vascular sources includes:

1. Coronary artery disease. Pain from coronary artery insufficiency (angina) and from infarction (ischemia) may be referred to the TMJ area. The most common site is the angle of the mandible. The mechanism for this referral is by the cervical internuncials which connect with cervical nerves 1 to 3. These nerves have neurons involved with the transmission of pain located in subnucleus caudalis (refer to section on the trigeminal nerve). The clinician should routinely consider coronary artery disease as a possible cause of MPD symptoms until eliminated by diagnostic procedures.
2. Temporal arteritis
3. Aneurysm (rare)
4. Pulseless disease
5. Migraine headaches
6. Cluster headaches

Pain in the dental-facial structure can be caused by:

1. Periodontal lesions
2. Pulpal pathologies
3. Caries
4. Sinusitis
5. Mucosal lesions
6. Facial dermatitis including herpetic lesions
7. Salivary gland pathology

The neural division includes pain from:

1. Peripheral overlappage of nerve fibers. Peripheral nerve fibers in the facial region display striking degrees of overlappage. Therefore, pathology in one area may cause

pain in a site removed from the origin of the pathology but innervated by an overlapping nerve fiber.

2. Idiopathic trigeminal neuralgia (tic douloureux). Idiopathic trigeminal neuralgia may be divided into typical and atypical forms. The primary features of the typical form are pain elicited by stimulating certain trigger areas, sharp, excruciating pain lasting usually several minutes, pain falling within the area innervated by the trigeminal nerve, or one-sided pain.[13(p71)]
3. Neurologic neoplasms.
4. Multiple sclerosis.

Pain of brainstem origin In this division is pain caused by brainstem synaptic overlappage. As has been noted, six different nerve trunks have neurons involved with the modality of pain located in the spinal nucleus of the trigeminal nerve. This central overlappage is a major source of referred pain.

Pain of cortical-thalamic origin Two types of pain are grouped in this division. The cortex, after perceiving the pain, evaluates it on the basis of locus, intensity, and past history of similar discomfort. There are internuncial connections with both the limbic system as well as return autonomic and effector centers. Thus, the cortex evokes an evaluative set of parameters in perceiving sensation. However, the discomfort perceived by the patient may be purely of cortical origin. That is, the pain is psychogenic and without any basis in actual pathology. There are many patients in whom the pain is both of pathologic and psychologic origin. Indeed, many of the patients whose discomfort is in the musculoskeletal area must be simultaneously treated for any demonstrable pathology and receive psychological or psychiatric support. A diagnosis of pure psychogenic distress should be made only after all diagnostic procedures have proven negative. This includes referral to a specialist in MPD, a neurologist, or a otolaryngologist if indicated.

The author has found that in those patients who can point to a specific small area as their major source of discomfort, a pathologic cause can almost invariably be discovered. Conversely, patients who describe broad areas of pain, especially if the areas of involvement cross the midline, often have a marked psychological aspect to their discomfort. There even have been cases reported of purely hysterical trismus.

Dental and facial pain, therefore, can arise from a number of loci. Regardless of the source, it has three components.

1. A motor component which produces grimacing, shoulder movements, alterations in salivary flow, eye movements, and respiratory and cardiovascular changes.
2. The awareness component which runs from the subnucleus

caudalis to the somatosensory areas I and II of the cortex. The pathway consists of heavily myelinated fibers which conduct rapidly and with great fidelity. There is only one synapse in this pathway. It is found in the ventral posteromedial (VPM) nucleus in the thalamus. This system makes us aware of the location, quality, and intensity of the pain.

3. The effect component. A third, ill-defined but identified pathway exists between the subnucleus caudalis and the limbic system. This pathway has many interconnections and is the area which generates an emotional response to the perceived pain.

Dental and facial pain, like pain from other areas of the body, is modulated by a gate-control mechanism as formulated by Melzack and Wall.[15]

Theories of Myofacial Pain Dysfunction

If the skeletal, traumatic, neurologic, neoplastic, and infectious causes of dentofacial pain are eliminated, there still remain 70% to 80% of patients presenting with MPD symptomatology. These are the patients with myospasm, trigger points, referred pain, occlusal disharmonies, and emotional stress patterns. The etiology of this MPD area and the appropriate treatment modes is at this time unresolved. However, several etiologic theories have evolved and most MPD specialists will be devotees of one of the major schools of thought.

Deboever[16] has categorized five major etiologic theories of myofacial pain dysfunction of the myospastic category, the mechanical displacement theory, the muscle theory, the neuromuscular theory, the psychophysiologic theory, and the psychologic theory.

Mechanical displacement theory This theory is based on the observation that some MPD patients have overclosure of the mandible. This may be caused by the loss of or improper eruption of the posterior dentition. The overclosure of the mandible is thought to place undue pressure on the auriculotemporal and chorda tympani nerves and the eustachian tube. Adherents of this theory place great emphasis on the visualization of equal anterior and posterior joint spaces on roentgenographic examination. The theory has been challenged on anatomic grounds.

Muscle theory The basis of this theory is muscle hyperactivity. The hyperactivity serves as an initiator of myospasm, which then spreads to its primary and secondary referred pain sites. Although there is no basis for refutation of this theory, the author believes that it is too narrow and does not take into account other viable aspects of the MPD problem.

Neuromuscular theory The neuromuscular theory is based on a functional disharmony between the occlusal interface and the desired muscle response. This interaction has been described previously in this chapter. The incompatibility leads to parafunctional habits such as grinding and clenching of the dentition (bruxing). The grinding and clenching may occur during the waking hours but is most often manifested during sleep. The bruxing habit leads to abnormal contractile states and, hence, myospastic activity. The theory covers many of the clinical MPD problems which are commonly seen and, indeed, may be the most popular theory. Its major defect is that it does not explain why many patients with abnormalities in the occlusal interface do not have MPD problems.

Psychologic and psychophysiologic theories The basis of these theories is that patients under stress have increased tension in the masticatory musculature.[17] Some supporters of this school believe that the syndrome is purely psychogenic and should be treated primarily from a psychoanalytic point of view.

Laskin[18] has evolved a psychophysiologic approach to MPD problems. This theory states that myospastic activity is the primary cause of MPD symptomatology. It is further believed that fatigue caused by tension-related oral habits is the major cause of the myospastic activity. The theory does take into account the necessity for physiologic harmony between the components of the stomatognathic system as well as the obvious influence that psychologic factors have in the MPD syndrome. At present, there are too few data to unequivocably support this theory.[19] However, the author believes that its multifactorial base is far more rational than the other existing theories of MPD dysfunction.

It can be stated that the myofacial aspect of the syndrome is multifactorial, and there can be little doubt that the emotional status of the patient is one of the most important of these factors. However, for any lasting improvement in the patient's symptoms, all of the components of the stomatognathic system must also be functioning within the physiologic parameters of that patient.

Myofacial pain dysfunction, therefore, has both a physical and emotional component. Both aspects of the problem must be accurately diagnosed and both must be treated. There can only be one accurate diagnosis, but any one of a number of treatment modes may be equally successful.

Conclusion

The exploration of myofacial pain dysfunction syndrome has revealed the complexities associated with this multifactorial entity. The material contained in this chapter should provide the reader with the basic information needed to intelligently evaluate, support, and refer for appropriate treatment those patients with possible MPD problems.

APPENDIX

SCREENING EXAMINATION FOR THE MYOFACIAL PAIN DYSFUNCTION SYNDROME

The following simple screening examination is presented as a guide for the physician.

History

A thorough and complete history is absolutely essential. It should include such questions as:

- When did the problem start? Probe the answer and *listen* to the responses. Was it associated with trauma? Dental treatment? Surgery? An emotionally stressful event?
- Do you find it difficult to open your mouth? Chew food? Find a comfortable jaw position?
- Has your mouth ever locked open?
- When is the pain worse? If upon awakening, it may indicate bruxing or clenching. If upon eating, it may indicate dental or salivary pathology. If it is progressive during the day, it may indicate neuromuscular problems.
- Do your jaws click?
- Ask "If I could relieve you of all symptoms on this appointment how would it change your life?" Answers such as, "I could get married, get a friend, etc," indicate psychologic involvement.[20]
- Is there a history of headache? Type? Duration? Severity? Possibility of migraine, cluster headache, Ménière's disease, CNS lesion, tension, MPD syndrome.
- Last, but most important: Where does it hurt? Those patients who point to a single spot or area almost invariably will have some demonstrable pathology as a cause of their discomfort. Those patients who trace a very broad area, especially if they cross the midline or are vague as to the exact locus of their discomfort, should be carefully evaluated as having a psychologic basis for their difficulty.

Observation of the Patient

- Is there facial asymmetry? May indicate muscular imbalance or tumor.
- Are the midlines of the upper and lower dentition congruent?

- Is there asymmetry in swallowing? An indication of neurologic pathology.
- Mandibular movement. Any patient should be able to place the first three fingers of their nondominant hand vertically between the maxillary and mandibular incisor teeth.
- Are there signs of excessive stress or nervousness?
- Are other body structures (shoulders, hips, or legs,) symmetrical or uneven?
- Does the mandible deviate to either side when opened? Indicates neuromuscular imbalance.

Physical Examination

- Otic. Does the patient complain of tinnitus, stuffiness, otic pain, some feelings of vertigo? Positive responses call for elimination of labyrinthitis, otitis, CNS lesions, and neuroses as diagnostic possibilities.
- Palpation should include the TMJ, both externally and intrameatally, masticatory musculature, submandibular areas, sternocleidomastoid, splenius capitus, trapezius, occipital areas, and shoulder areas. Palpation of the musculature should be performed with the mouth held open.
- Check for lymphadenopathy.
- Joint function. Place a stethoscope along a line from the tragus of the ear to the ala of the nose, about 1.5 to 2.5 cm anterior to the tragus. Ask the patient to open and close the mouth slowly. Is a click present? Is there crepitus? Clicks usually indicate incoordinated neuromuscular activity. Crepitus could be indicative of arthritic changes.

Evaluation

- Every patient must be considered an individual and unique challenge. Do not categorize your patient.
- Rule out by diagnostic results other systemic disease possibilities including otic and labyrinthine disorders, neurologic disorders, neoplasms, traumas, and vascular and cardiac sources.
- If these systemic pathologies have been eliminated, and clicks, myospasm, limited mandibular motion, and preauricular pain are present, singly or in any combination, then MPD should be considered as a prime diagnosis. The patient should then be referred to an MPD specialist or MPD clinic for further evaluation and treatment.

The author wishes to thank the following staff members of the University of Maryland School of Dentistry: Dr. Robert Bennett of the Department of Physiology for his modifications to the myospastic cycle diagram, Dr. Daniel Overholser, Chairman of the Department of Oral Diagnosis, and Dr. Antoinette Balciunas, of the same department, for their review of this chapter and their helpful critique and suggestions.

REFERENCES

1. Zarb GA, Carlsson GE: *Temporo-Mandibular Joint Function and Dysfunction*. St Louis, CV Mosby, 1979, pp 175–189.
2. Shore NA: *Temporo-Mandibular Joint Dysfunction and Occlusal Equilibration,* ed 2. Philadelphia, Lippincott, 1976.
3. Burch J: *Anat Rec* 1966;156:433–437.
4. Solberg WK, Clark GT: *Temporo-Mandibular Joint Problems.* Chicago, Quintessence, 1980, pp 33–42.
5. Wyke B: The neurology of joints. *Ann R Coll Surg Engl* 1967;41:25–50.
6. Davies PL: Electromyographic study of superficial neck muscles in mandibular function. *J Dent Res* 1979;58:1.
7. Marbach JJ, Lipton JA: The relation of diagnosis to treatment in the facial pain patient. *NY State Dent J* 1977;43:282.
8. Guyton AC: *Basic Human Physiology*. Philadelphia, WB Saunders, 1977.
9. Morgan HM, Hall WP, Vamus JS: *Diseases of the Temporo-Mandibular Apparatus.* St Louis, CV Mosby 1977, pp 26–35.
10. Travell JG: Myofacial trigger points: Clinical view, in Bonica JJ, Albe-Sessard D (eds): *Advances in Pain Research and Therapy.* New York, Raven Press, 1976, vol 1, pp 919–926.
11. Ramsey WO, Staling LM: Palpation of the Musculature of the Masticatory System. ILC Physiology, Baltimore, University of Maryland School of Dentistry 1978, p 354.
12. Dubner R, Sessle B, Storey A: *The Neural Basis of Oral and Facial Function.* New York, Plenum Press, 1978.
13. Alling CC III, Mahan PE: *Facial Pain,* ed 2. Philadelphia, Lea and Febiger, 1977, pp 25–41.
14. Roberts A, Pierson D: Etiology and treatment of idiopathic trigeminal and atypical facial neuralgias. *J Oral Surg Oral Med Oral Pathol* 1979; 48:298–310.
15. Melzack R, Wall PD: Pain mechanisms: A New Theory. *Science* 1965; 150:971–978.
16. Deboever J: Functional disturbances of the temporomandibular joints. *Oral Sci Rev* 1973;2:100.
17. Thomas LJ, Tiber N, Schireson S: The effects of anxiety and frustration on muscular tension related to the temporo-mandibular joint syndrome. *Oral Surg* 1973;36:763.
18. Laskin DM: Etiology of the pain dysfunction syndrome, *J Am Dent Assoc* 1969;79:147.
19. Gutto R, Spektor M: TMJ dysfunction: Etiology, diagnosis, treatment, review of literature. *J Am Coll Dent* 1981;29:3.
20. Scheman P, Freese A: *Management of TMJ Problems.* St Louis, CV Mosby, 1962.

SECTION V
Drugs

16 Nonsteroidal Anti-Inflammatory Drugs

Andrew R. Klipper
A. Lewis Kolodny

Adequate management of the patient with rheumatic complaints necessitates an understanding that we are addressing over 100 different disorders and diseases. Obviously, determination of proper diagnosis may bring about more specific treatment. Indeed, proper therapy often involves a multidisciplinary approach with cooperative efforts of primary physician, rheumatologist, physiatrist, orthopedist, plastic surgeon, psychiatrist, physical therapist, occupational therapist, nurse specialist, and social worker. Nevertheless, the initial impetus for the patient to seek care from the physician is pain. The evolution of the medical profession occurred because of this fact, with early man approaching the shaman, the witch doctor, for alleviation of pain.

Unfortunately, early measures directed at pain relief involved opiates, first in crude form and later in more purified drugs. Subsequently, salicylates appeared on the scene and in the past 25 years or so a number of nonnarcotic analgesics, which contributed a modicum of pain relief but, nevertheless, did not represent a panacea. Further problems included the pessimistic attitude displayed by both physician and the suffering patient. As our understanding of the constant feedback of psyche and soma in modifying pain perception became clarified, treatment of acute and chronic pain drew closer to success.

Recent advances and understanding of neuropathology and neurophysiology have allowed the pharmacologist to approach management of pain with a more scientific and less empirical attitude. Even so, empirical prescribing of drugs becomes necessary until specific etiologies are established for all of the multifaceted rheumatologic complaints. When that utopian day arrives, the clinicians may then direct their energies toward removing the etiologic causes of pain, and thus stop pain before it occurs, or at least relieve pain in its early stages. Today, in a few instances, this is possible.

The development of nonsteroidal anti-inflammatory drugs (NSAIDs) during the last two decades represents a major contribution to the therapy of both acute and chronic pain in rheumatic disease. Unlike the action of central-acting analgesics without anti-inflammatory effects, this new group of pain-relieving drugs offers notable reduction of inflammation by influencing the prostaglandin system. Hence, the role of nonsteroidal anti-inflammatory drugs in treating the 100 or more rheumatic disorders is important.

Historically, analgesic and antipyretic effects of salicylates have been known from the time of the ancient Greeks. Aspirin was first developed by Von Gerhardt in 1853, but only after Bayer Pharmaceutical Company succeeded in synthesizing this agent in 1893 was aspirin brought into general use as an analgesic, antipyretic, and later anti-inflammatory agent.

Subsequently, the para-aminophenol group of drugs was studied including phenylacetamide (acetanilid), acetophenetidin (phenacetin), and acetaminophen (Tylenol, Tempra, paracetamol). This group of drugs lacked the anti-inflammatory effects of aspirin and, hence, had limited use in inflammatory rheumatic disease. Moreover, the toxicity of this series of drugs, with the exception of acetaminophen, limited their use. However, acetaminophen has been used as an aspirin substitute with effective noninflammatory analgesic action. In addition, acetaminophen has an antipyretic action. Its action is peripheral. Although large doses are hepatotoxic, its lack of gastric irritation offers advantages over aspirin usage, provided the anti-inflammatory effects are not important. As yet, the nephrotoxic reaction of its parent chemical is not fully accepted, but recent work indicates a strong suspicion that acetaminophen may produce nephrotoxicity. Acetaminophen blocks prostaglandin synthesis centrally, accounting for its antipyretic effects. However, its lack of peripheral antiprostaglandin effect may account for its failure to block inflammation.

Comprising a group of useful but toxic agents, the pyrazolines are no longer in general use except for phenylbutazone (Butazolidin, Azolid-A). This class of drugs causes a potent anti-inflammatory response with less analgesic effect in noninflammatory conditions. Prolonged usage in large dose is limited by its hematologic toxicity. Gastric irritation and salt and fluid retention are commonly seen. Oxyphenbutazone (Tandearil), a parahydroxy analog of phenylbutazone, offers similar pharmacologic action and side effects. Usual dosage is 100 mg given four times a day. If no response is noted within one week, the drug should be discontinued. We have used 100 to 200 mg daily in long-term therapy in treating ankylosing spondylitis with a minimum of side effects.

A number of centrally acting nonnarcotic synthetic analgesics without anti-inflammatory effects have been described during the past two decades. Among these was ethoheptazine citrate (Zactane), a congener of mepiridine. Lacking the addicting properties of mepiridine, Zactane also lacked the analgesic potency of its parent drug. Propoxyphene (Darvon) was in wide use as an analgesic agent without addicting qualities. Derived from methadone, it is now classified as a possible addicting agent. Again, it offers no antipyretic or anti-inflammatory actions. Its potency as a central acting analgesic resembles that of codeine. Pentazocine (Talwin) is a centrally acting agonist-antagonist narcotic, with no anti-inflammatory effect. Central nervous system side effects including dysphoria plus potential tolerance and habituation limit its use. Other agonist-antagonist narcotics available for parenteral use will not be discussed in this chapter. Neither will the use of narcotics be presented.

In 1963, a new potent nonsteroidal anti-inflammatory analgesic, indomethacin (Indocin) was described as a valuable tool in treating rheumatic disease. Chemically, a serotonin-related drug, it was known as 1-(p-chlorbenzoyl)-5 methoxy-2-methyl indole-3-acetic acid. Its value as a potent analgesic in rheumatic disease is limited by its central nervous system (CNS) side effects and gastric toxicity. Nevertheless, in a dosage of 25 to 50 mg four times a day, this drug is still widely used despite the competition of the newer nonsteroidal anti-inflammatory analgesics. It is well-confirmed that both aspirin and indomethacin inhibit the transformation of arachnidonic acid to stable prostaglandins. These two agents, plus all of the nonsteroidal anti-inflammatory analgesics which we will describe, probably reduce pain and inflammation by inhibiting prostaglandin biosynthesis by affecting the enzyme, cyclo-oxygenase, which produces the cyclic-endoperoxides from arachnidonic acid, thus reducing this mediator of inflammation. Indomethacin may also increase intracellular cyclic adenosinemonophosphate (AMF), which may inhibit inflammation.

The appearance of numerous nonsteroidal anti-inflammatory analgesics offers the clinician a most useful group of nonspecific but effective pain relievers. Indeed, these drugs not only offer symptomatic relief, but help bring about suppression if not remission of inflammatory rheumatic disorders.

Ibuprofen (Motrin), one of many propionic acid derivatives, was the first of this new group of agents available in the United States since indomethacin. In clinical use for 15 years, doses of 1.2 to 1.6 g daily in four divided doses offer analgesic effect with mild anti-inflammatory action. In doses of 2.4 to 3.2 g daily, considerably more anti-inflammatory and analgesic effects are noted. Primary side effects consist of gastric irritation and rashes. Adverse gastric reactions represent half those seen in aspirin or indomethacin-treated patients. Less frequently found, indeed—much rarer reactions involving the CNS such as dizziness, headaches, and amblyopia-scotomata, and hematologic side effects, have been described. Also noted have been adverse hepatic reactions. On rare occasion, azotemia has been noted. Exacerbation of renal failure probably occurs through the inhibition of renal prostaglandins. A lupus erythematosus-like syndrome has been noted, as has a serum sickness allergic reaction.

Another of the profens, the propionic acid derivatives, is fenoprofen (Nalfon). Dosage of this drug varies from 600 to 3200 mg daily and is administered four times a day before meals. Analgesic effects are seen much sooner than anti-inflammatory action. Untoward reactions consisting of gastric toxicity are not common, and may occur in less than 2% of the patients. Adverse dermatologic reactions are noted in 1% of patients. However, 15% of persons receiving fenprofen have developed CNS side effects including dizziness, insomnia, tremor, or confusion.

Among the newer propionic acid derivatives is naproxen (Naprosyn). Because of its long half-life, 13 hours, it may be prescribed twice a day. Dosage ranging from 500 to 1000 mg daily is optimum. Most frequent adverse effects are gastrointestinal, including peptic ulcer. Rashes, headaches, dizziness, visual disturbances, and tinnitus are among the more frequent adverse reactions noted in over 1% of patients.

In the latter part of 1960, a new series of pyrole acetic acid derivatives were developed. Tolmetin (Tolectin), one of this group, is related to indomethacin, by substituting pyrole for the indole nucleus of indomethacin. We find 800 to 1800 mg a day divided in four doses offers best therapeutic response. However, on occasion, 2000 mg a day has been given. Gastrointestinal side effects are the most common of the adverse reactions presented. Other untoward reactions include headaches, dizziness, rashes, and fluid retention.

Although most of the nonsteroidal anti-inflammatory analgesic agents interfere with the use of warfarin compounds and may, indeed, increase bleeding when given simultaneously, tolmetin does not seem to offer as much danger when simultaneous use of both of these drugs are given.

More recently, a related compound, zomepirac (Zomax) has been released. This indene derivative has been shown to have potent analgesic effect and anti-inflammatory action. In doses of 100 mg four times a day, it offers a useful addition to the armamentarium of anti-inflammatory analgesics. Side effects of gastrointestinal irritation and rash are the most common adverse reactions. Other untoward effects are similar to those of previously described nonsteroidal anti-inflammatory drugs.

In 1972, an analog of indomethacin, sulindac (Clinoril), was described. An indene structure was substituted for the indole ring of indomethacin. The potency of sulindac as an anti-inflammatory analgesic was comparable to the effects of its parent drug, indomethacin. Moreover, the CNS and gastrointestinal untoward side effects of indomethacin were decreased with use of sulindac. The mean half-life of sulindac is 7.8 hr, and that of its active sulfide metabolite is 16.4 hr, thus allowing a twice-a-day dosage. In a dosage of 200 to 400 mg daily, its effectiveness is that of 2400 to 4800 mg of aspirin. Adverse reactions include gastrointestinal symptoms, rashes, dizziness, headaches, nervousness, tinnitus, and edema.

Table 16-1
Nonsteroidal Anti-inflammatory Analgesics (NSAID)

Salicylates
- aspirin
- magnesium salicylate
- choline magnesium salicylate
- salsalate
- diflunisal

Pyrazolines
- phenylbutazone
- azapropazone

Indole Acetic Acid Derivative
- indomethacin

Indene Acetic Acid Derivatives
- sulindac
- zomepirac

Pyrole Acetic Acid Derivative
- tolmetin

Phenyl Acetic Acid Derivative
- diclofenac

Propionic Acid Derivatives
- ibuprofen
- fenoprofen
- naproxen
- fenbufen
- ketoprofen
- pirprofen
- oxaprozin
- benoxaprofen

Anthranilic Acid Derivative
- meclofenamet

Benzothiazine Derivative
- piroxicam

Quinazolinone, Nonorganic Acid Derivative
- proquazone

Derived from mefenamic acid, an analgesic marred by side effects of colitis is meclofenamat (Meclomen), one of the anthranilic acid series. In doses of 200 to 400 mg given three to four times a day, it offers potent analgesic and anti-inflammatory actions. A dual anti-inflammatory action is postulated, both by inhibition of prostaglandin synthesis and by its ability to compete for binding at the prostaglandin binding site. Col itis, with diarrhea and cramps apparently caused by metabolite, is fairly common. However, we have found that a bulk laxative such as Metamucil given prophylactically once a week or three to four times a day therapeutically affords relief from this reversible problem. Peptic ulcer disease is uncommon. Rashes, headaches, dizziness, and tinnitus represent other more commonly described side effects.

Many other nonsteroidal anti-inflammatory analgesics are available in Europe and other parts of the world. A number of these are being studied in the United States and, assuming proven efficacy and safety, several of these drugs will be available during the next five years. Among these is fenbufen, a propionic acid series derivative. Our studies have shown that adverse effects were reasonably few, with a high ratio of efficacy. Soon to be released is piroxicam (Feldene), a benzothiazine derivative, having advantages of compliance through a once-daily dose. Another of the profen group available in many countries but not released in the United States is ketoprofen. Clinical properties of this agent resemble those of naproxen.

Another of the propionic acid series that may be released in the country is oxaprozin. In double-blind studies, Kolodny and Klipper have noted marked efficacy with the usual untoward effects of this group of drugs. Soon to be available in the United States is pirprofen (Rengasil), a member of the propionic acid series. Klipper and Kolodny, among others, described its efficacy in osteoarthritis and rheumatoid arthritis. Proquazone represents an exception to the organic acid characteristics of NSAIDs. It has not been released but displays anti-inflammatory, analgesic effects. Side effects of diarrhea in some patients has presented a problem. As yet, this drug is not available in this country. Now being studied in the United States is diclofenac (Voltaren). This agent, a phenylacetic acid derivative, has been used in Europe with potent anti-inflammatory and analgesic effects. Other interesting NSAIDs under clinical investigation in this country include etodolic acid and isoxepac (Artil), an organic acid derivative.

Recently released in the United States by the FDA and subsequently withdrawn is a new profen derivative, benoxaprofen (Oraflex). This drug, unlike other NSAIDs, is a weak inhibitor of prostaglandin synthetase. Instead, this agent inhibits the lipoxygenase pathway of arachidonic acid metabolism and, in so doing, inhibits the formation of leukotrienes. Leukotrienes are patent mediators of inflammation. Furthermore, benoxaprofen inhibits mononuclear cell migration, thus reducing inflammation.

Since the half-life of benoxaprofen is 30 hours, the drug may be administered orally once a day in a dosage of 600 mg. Phototoxicity and onycholysis represent significant side effects, which can be prevented by sunscreen lotions and opaque nail polish. Gastrointestinal side effects and cholestasis with jaundice have been reported to occur in the elderly.

In considering usage of the NSAIDs, the question arises as to which drug is the most efficacious. One can only say that, despite a host of clinical studies, the final conclusion is that some patients respond better to one agent than another. Assuming adequate amounts are prescribed for the individual, if one of the NSAIDs fails to offer relief, another should be tried. While such trials seem to present an unscientific approach, indeed, trial-and-error methodology is often used in therapeutics. Another serious consideration is the fact that in aspirin-sensitive patients, particularly those with nasal polyps and asthma, the use of NSAIDs may be hazardous with severe allergic reactions.

A number of interactions involving nonsteroidal anti-inflammatory drugs have been described. There are a number of studies that indicate that the use of aspirin concomitantly with indomethacin may decrease the efficacy of the indomethacin and the aspirin. There are others, however, which have found that, despite the fact that aspirin and indomethacin seem to compete with the binding of serum protein, the two together become somewhat additive in efficacy.

There seems to be some interaction between aspirin and ibuprofen. By the same token, prescribing aspirin and ibuprofen together in some patients seems to produce a greater anti-inflammatory response than one would expect with the single drug.

In studying a number of the other nonsteroidal anti-inflammatory analgesics, similar findings seem to be present. For example, administration of naproxen to patients receiving aspirin seems to increase plasma clearance of naproxen. Acetaminophen, when administered with tolmetin, apparently increased analgesic efficacy. Tolmetin levels in the plasma do not appear to be reduced by aspirin. By the same token, acetaminophen apparently reduces anti-inflammatory effects of indomethacin. A number of other drugs that reportedly antagonize the anti-inflammatory action of indomethacin include chlorpromazine, protriptyline, and d-proproxyphene.

There still seems to be a great deal of difference in thought among various investigators whether these facts are clinically important. Our personal feelings are not to use two anti-inflammatory agents simultaneously because of the possibility of inducing peptic ulcer disease. However, controlled studies confirming this fact are not available. There are a number of rheumatologists who think that using two nonsteroidal anti-inflammatory analgesics simultaneously may permit smaller dosage of each and increase of analgesic anti-inflammatory efficacy, with no increase in untoward effects. Certainly at this time, until further data are available, the clinician should be conservative in his approach using more than one anti-inflammatory drug.

Because of the known efficacy of aspirin, which, unfortunately, presents gastric problems in many patients, a number of salicylates have been developed in recent years, presumably with the analgesic, anti-inflammatory effects of aspirin, but with decreased ulcerogenic adverse effects. Enteric-coated aspirin (Ecotrin), when absorbed, certainly fits safety criteria. However, salicylate levels must be monitored to assure adequate absorption. Among the newer salicylates are salsalate (Disalcid), magnesium salicylate (Magan), and choline-magnesium salicylate (Trilisate). These non-acetylated salicylates offer less possibility of gastric irritation and no effect on normal platelet function. Inhibition of prothrombin synthesis in the liver with prolongation of the prothrombin time may occur with aspirin and with most of the nonsteroidal anti-inflammatory analgesics, except possibly tolmetin. Adequate salicylate levels are achieved with the use of these newer salicylates. There are those, however, who feel that the acetylated salicylate, such as aspirin, offers more efficacy. Whether this is factual or not is unknown at this time.

Another salicylate related nonsteroidal anti-inflammatory analgesic recently made available is diflunisal (Dolobid). This drug is a prostaglandin synthetase inhibitor with analgesic effects similar to acetaminophen, 600 mg, with codeine, 60 mg.

Diflunisal is not metabolized to salicylic acid but forms two soluble glucuronide conjugates. Hence, it differs from other salicylates. Its prolonged half-life of eight to ten hours permits a twice a day dosage. A loading dose of 1000 mg is followed by 500 mg twice a day.

Gastrointestinal side effects represent up to 8.7% of toxicity. Rash, dizziness, headache, tinnitus, and fatigue are the less prominent untoward effects.

While the use of the nonspecific nonsteroidal anti-inflammatory agents is widespread through a whole spectrum of rheumatic diseases and disorders, there are a few entities in which they have more specific therapeutic effect. Among these are gold compounds, which must be administered parenterally. These include gold sodium thiomalate (Myochrysine) and aurothioglucose (Solganal). It is known that, very shortly, an oral form of gold (Auranofin) will be available. Gold is used in treating rheumatoid arthritis and psoriatic arthritis. Another agent of the slow-acting variety that is used in treating rheumatoid arthritis is penicillamine. Furthermore, an antimalarial drug, hydroxychloroquine (Plaquenil), has been useful in treating both rheumatoid arthritis and some of the manifestations of systemic lupus erythematosus. However, it is not the purpose of this chapter to discuss these drugs in detail.

When considering the treatment of gout in its chronic form, the use of agents to reduce uric acid levels is most helpful. We will only mention them by name briefly. These include probenecid (Benemid), sulfinpyrazone (Anturane), and allopurinol (Zyloprim). Again, the details of these drugs will not be discussed within the scope of this chapter.

The search continues for better and safer nonsteroidal anti-inflammatory agents. Until curative agents are available for the 100 or more rheumatic complaints that have been described, we must continue to depend upon the supportive effect of these useful drugs.

BIBLIOGRAPHY

Ambanell A: A multiclinic study in osteoarthritis. *Eur J Rheumatol Inflammation* 1978;1:45–46.

Beavers WT: Interaction of narcotics and mood-altering drugs: A brief historical review. Recent studies on the nature and management of acute pain. *Hosp Pract* (special report), Jan 1976;8–13.

Brooks PM, Hill W, Geddes R, et al: Diclofenac and ibuprofen in rheumatoid arthritis and osteoarthritis. *Med J Aust* 1980;67:29.

Calabro JJ: Long-term reappraisal of indomethacin. *Drug Ther* 1975;5:46–47, 51–54,59–60.

Castles JJ, Moore TL, Vaughan JH, et al: Multicenter comparison of naproxen and indomethacin in rheumatoid arthritis. *Arch Intern Med* 1978; 138:362–366.

Chalem F, Pena M, Lizarazo H, et al: Comparison of fenbufen and aspirin in the treatment of rheumatoid arthritis. *Curr Ther Res* 1977;22:769–783.

Ehrlich GE, Roth S: Rheumatoid arthritis, long-term therapy with tolmetin sodium. *Orthop Dig* 1976;4:16–18,21–24.

Higgs GA, Moncada S, Vane JR, et al: The mode of action of anti-inflammatory drugs which prevent the peroxidation of arachidonic acid. *Clin Rheumat Dis* 1980;5:675–693.

Huskisson EC: Classification of anti-rheumatic drugs. *Clin Rheumat Dis* 1979; 5:353–357.

Kantor TG: A double blind evaluation of the efficacy and safety of proquazone compared to aspirin in patients with osteoarthritis. Presented at the Fourteenth International Congress of Rheumatology, San Francisco, June-July 1977.

Kantor TG: Analgesics for arthritis. *Clin Rheumat Dis* 1980;5:525–531.

Kantor TG: Studies of orally administered narcotics, ataractics, and combination of the two. *Hosp Pract* (special report), Jan 1976;8–13.

Klipper AR, Kolodny AL: Pirprofen in treatment of osteoarthritis. Presented at the Fifteenth International Congress of Rheumatology, Paris, 1981.

Kolodny AL, McLoughlin PT: *Comprehensive Approach to Therapy of Pain.* Springfield, IL, Charles C Thomas, 1966.

Lee P, Anderson JA, Miller J, et al: Evaluation of analgesic action and efficacy of antirheumatic drugs. *J Rheumatol* 1976;3:283.

Rodvein R, Cooke AR: Aspirin revisited in Jensen KG, Killman S (eds): *Antiplatelet Drugs and Thrombosis.* Copenhagen, Munksgaard, 1976, pp 141–150.

Zizic TM, Sutton JD, Stevens MB: Piroxicam and osteoarthritis: A controlled study. *R Soc Med* 1:71–82.

17 Opioid Receptors and Peptides in Pain Control

Michael J. Kuhar

The utilization of morphine for control of pain is one of the most important tools that a physician possesses. In the last few years, hallmark discoveries have been made in the basic sciences which help us understand how the body generates, processes, and controls painful stimuli. The goal of this chapter is to summarize recent advances in pharmacology and anatomy related to how opiate drugs produce analgesia.

In order to understand how the opiate drugs are involved in the control of pain, we must first summarize certain anatomical features involved in the transmission of pain. Painful stimuli are carried through the peripheral nerves to the central nervous system via small, unmyelinated fibers in the dorsal roots. A key place for the integration of nociceptive stimuli is the substantia gelatinosa of the spinal cord. Other key areas include the raphe nuclei of the medulla, the floor of the fourth ventricle, the midbrain periaqueductal grey, and the dorsal medial thalamus. The involvement of these latter areas in pain transmission is evident from a number of experiments showing that direct stimulation or implantation of drugs in these areas result in a profound analgesia without general behavioral depression.[1-4] This chapter will discuss the experimental evidence showing that these anatomical areas contain high concentrations of opiate receptors as well as the enkephalins.

The concept that drugs act at specific molecular sites in the body, hereafter referred to as receptors, to elicit specific biochemical, behavioral, and physiological effects has long been recognized in pharmacology and physiology. The evolution of the notion of receptors and the methods designed for studying specific receptors in tissues have been steadily refined over the past decade. Studies by Pert and Snyder,[5] Terenius,[6] and Simon and co-workers[7] succeeded in identifying the opiate receptor in nervous tissues. Once the methods existed for identifying these specific opiate receptors in the body, it was possible to study their distribution as well as more subtle aspects of the mechanisms of opiate drug action. This chapter will stress the distribution of opiate receptors and its relationship to pain.

At the present time, a discussion of opiate drugs would be incomplete without mention of the enkephalins which, all evidence indicates, are the naturally occurring factors that normally utilize the opiate receptors. The discovery of the enkephalins so soon after the identification of opiate receptors is one of the most interesting stories in science. Since the body does not normally contain opiate drugs like morphine, it has always been a puzzle as to why the body would have specific receptors for the drug. It certainly seemed feasible that the receptors existed for some other naturally occurring biochemical phenomenon. This possibility, as well as certain experiments, led scientists to search for endogenous factors which were morphine-like in that they acted at the specific receptors. Hughes,[8] working with bioassays developed by Kosterlitz for opiate drugs, was able to identify a factor in pig brain which appeared to be an endogenous opioid. Subsequent purification and chemical analysis of this factor indicated the presence of two peptides called leucine-enkephalin and methionine-enkephalin.[9] Their amino acid sequences are tyr-gly-gly-phe-leu and tyr-gly-gly-phe-met, respectively. Once the chemical structures of these factors were known, it was possible to synthesize these peptides and, by appropriate procedures, raise antibodies to these peptides. These antibodies can be used in both radioimmunoassay as well as in immunohistochemical procedures to localize enkephalin in the nervous system. This chapter will also summarize available information on this distribution as it applies to mechanisms of pain.

The Opiate Receptors

By utilizing the techniques for identifying the opiate receptor in neuronal tissue, investigators examined the distribution of opiate receptors in the various regions of the monkey and human brain.[10,11] These studies showed that the content of opiate receptors varied markedly in the various brain regions. As suspected, there were elevated levels of receptors in areas associated with pain, such as the dorsomedial thalamus and periaqueductal grey of the midbrain. But, interestingly, other areas of the brain had elevated levels as well (Table 17-1). For example, various portions of the limbic system, a system in the brain associated with emotionality, also had high levels. Perhaps these receptors mediate the euphoria caused by opiates. Thus, opiate receptors were found in areas associated with painful stimuli, but they were also found in other areas which is consistent with observations that opiates affect a wide variety of bodily processes aside from pain.[12-14]

Table 17-1
Regional Distribution of Enkephalin in Monkey Brain*

Region	Enkephalin concentration (Units/mg protein)	Opiate receptor density (fmole stereospecific [^{3}H] dihydromorphine bound/mg protein)
Precentral gyrus	0.41 ± 0.07	3.4
Temporal pole	0.36 ± 0.07	
Frontal pole	0.35 ± 0.04	11.9
Occipital pole	0.24 ± 0.04	2.3
Hippocampus	0.52 ± 0.07	12.5
Anterior hypothalamus	4.20 ± 0.47	24.3
Posterior hypothalamus	1.35 ± 0.11	24.7
Medial thalamus	0.57 ± 0.04	24.6
Lateral thalamus	0.25 ± 0.02	7.8
Periaqueductal grey	1.48 ± 0.16	31.1
Raphe area	1.08 ± 0.06	8.2
Floor of fourth ventricle	1.14 ± 0.08	6.3
Spinal cord (cervical)		
Dorsal cord (white and grey)	0.72	3.1 (White)
Ventral cord (white and grey)	0.72	3.3 (White)

*Data are expressed as mean values ± SEM from three different experiments.[25]

The interesting results obtained in these biochemical studies prompted the utilization of high resolution light microscopic methods for localizing opiate receptors in sections of brain tissue. Kuhar[15-17] developed such a method for localizing cholinergic muscarinic receptors in brain, and it was applied to the question of where opiate receptors were localized. The earliest experiments confirmed and extended the biochemical studies on human and monkey material. There were high densities of opiate receptors in the substantia gelatinosa of the spinal cord (see Figure 17-1). There were also elevated densities in the substantia gelatinosa of the spinal trigeminal nucleus, an area concerned with processing painful stimuli from the region of the head. The periaqueductal grey and floor of the fourth ventricle also had elevated levels of opiate receptors. In addition, the dorsal medial nucleus of the thalamus showed elevated densities of opiate receptors as did the so-called "intralaminar nuclei" of the thalamus. Thus, these light microscopic studies revealed high levels of opiate receptors at several places in the brain known to be involved in the control of painful stimuli.[12-14] Thus, it seems likely that opiate drugs affect the process of pain at several levels in the brain.

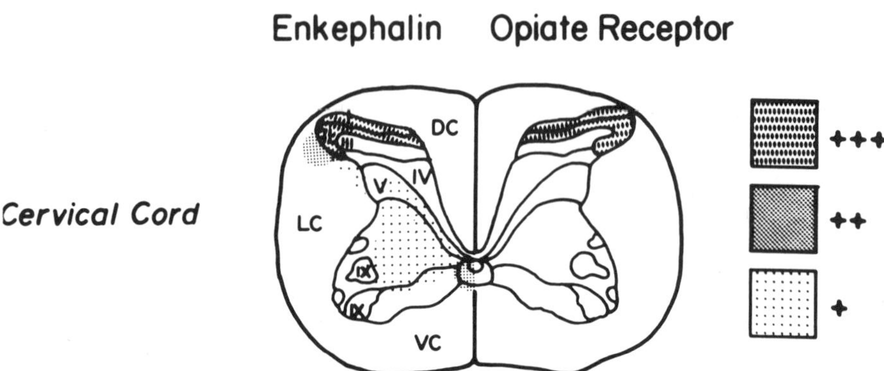

Figure 17-1 Schematic localization of enkephalins (left side) and opiate receptors (right side) in cervical spinal cord. A high density of both enkephalins and opiate receptors was found in laminae I and II (substantia gelatinosa). From Atweh and Kuhar[13] and Uhl et al.[19] Reprinted with permission.

Recent experiments indicate that opiates are probably most sensitive at supraspinal sites. In animal preparations where the spinal cord has been severed, it takes much higher doses of opiates to suppress painful reflexes than it does in an intact animal. This suggests that the first site that opiates act is above the spinal cord, while at higher doses they can effectively inhibit pain at the level of the spinal cord.[1] Among the important supraspinal sites are the medullary raphe nuclei which contain serotonin and which also appear to have adjacent to them enkephalin-containing cells.[18]

The Opioid Peptides Enkephalins

While there are a numer of peptides that appear to have opioid-like or morphine-like activity,[19-21] the peptides that shall be discussed here are the enkephalins. It is thought that these are the endogenous factors affecting opiate receptors in the brain while other morphine-like peptides and proteins are of importance outside the central nervous system. Like the opiate receptors, the distribution of enkephalins varies markedly throughout the brain in biochemical studies (Table 1). These findings prompted the utilization of light microscopic techniques to localize the peptide with greater precision.

By using immunocytochemical methods, several laboratories have identified neurons in the central nervous system that contain the enkephalins. These neurons and their processes are found in areas mentioned above that contain opiate receptors. For example, the substantia gelatinosa contains axons, nerve terminals, and cell bodies that contain enkephalins (see Figure 1). The other areas in the brain which are involved in analgesia, such as the dorsal medial thalamus, also have enkephalin-containing neurons and processes. In further agreement with the studies on receptors, the enkephalins were found in other brain areas associated with other physiological functions known to be altered by opiates. But a striking result of these studies of enkephalins was that many of the areas with high levels of opiate receptors showed similarly high levels of enkephalins.[18,22-23] This coincident distribution of opiate receptors and enkephalins, as well as other experiments showing that opiate drug and enkephalins have similar actions, strongly support the notion that the enkephalins are the endogenous substrates of the opiate receptors. It is reasonable to assume that enkephalins function as neurotransmitters.[24,25]

The discovery of specific neuroanatomical systems related to pain is likely to rationalize and possibly revolutionize the physiological and surgical approaches to the control of pain. Also, the discovery that endogenously occurring peptides are involved in pain regulation opens a new area for pharmacological investigation.

Conclusions

All of the available data obtained in the past few years suggest the following model. Administration of opiate drugs results in the interactions of these drugs with specific membrane-bound receptors in various regions of the brain. These interactions result in specific alterations in the firing rates of the involved neurons. The receptors are normally utilized by pentapeptides released from nerve terminals as part of normal neuronal activity. These pentapeptides are likely to be neurotransmitter substances conceptually very similar in action to acetylcholine and norepinephrine. Since the enkephalin-containing systems and the related opioid receptors are concentrated in areas of the brain involved in the integration and transmission of painful information and stimuli, administration of opioid drugs has a profound suppression of painful stimuli. The discovery of these endogenous systems containing opioid peptides raises many new important questions. Can we find some way to alter the function of enkephalin-containing neurons without using opiate drugs? Is it possible to do this in such a way as to prevent addiction? Also, perhaps one can design peptides or drugs which may be lacking in many of the addiction liabilities of the opiate drugs. In any case, while there have been dramatic advances in this area in the last few years, this remarkable story continues to evolve and present new hopes and vistas for the control of pain.

REFERENCES

1. Basbaum AI, Fields HL: Endogenous pain control mechanisms: Review and hypothesis. *Ann Neurol* 1978;4:451–462.
2. Fields HL, Basbaum AI: Brainstem control of spinal pain transmission neurons. *Ann Rev Physiol* 1978;40:193–221.
3. Kerr FWL: Neuroanatomical substrates of nociception in the spinal cord. *Pain* 1975;1:325–356.
4. Melzack R: *The Puzzle of Pain.* New York, Basic Books Inc 1973.
5. Pert CB, Snyder SH: Properties of opiate receptor binding in rat brain. *Proc Natl Acad Sci* USA 1973;70:2243–2247.
6. Terenius L: Characteristics of the "receptor" for narcotic analgesics in synaptic plasma membrane fraction from rat brain. *Acta Pharmacol* 1973;33:377–384.
7. Simon EJ, Hiller JM, Edelmann I: Stereospecific binding of the potent narcotic analgesic (^3H) etorphine to rat-brain homogenate. *Proc Natl Acad Sci* USA 1973;70:1947–1949.
8. Hughes J: Isolation of an endogenous compound from the brain with pharmacological properties similar to morphine. *Brain Res* 1975;88:295–308.
9. Hughes J, Smith TW, Kosterlitz HW, et al: Identification of two related pentapeptides from the brain with potent opiate agonist activity. *Nature* 1975;258:577–579.
10. Kuhar MJ, Pert CB, Snyder SH: Regional distribution of opiate receptor binding in monkey and human brain. *Nature* 1973;245:447–450.
11. Hiller JM, Pearson J, Simon EJ: Distribution of stereo-specific binding of the potent narcotic analgesic etorphine in the human brain. Predominance in the limbic system. *Res Commun Chem Pathol Pharmacol* 1973;6:1052–1061.
12. Atweh SF, Kuhar MJ: Autoradiographic localization of opiate receptors in rat brain. I. The spinal cord and lower medulla. *Brain Res* 1977;124:53–68.
13. Atweh SF, Kuhar MJ: Autoradiographic localization of opiate receptors in rat brain. II. The brainstem. *Brain Res* 1977;129:1–12.
14. Atweh SF, Kuhar MJ: Autoradiographic localization of opiate receptors in rat brain. III. The telencephalon. *Brain Res* 1977;134:393–405.
15. Kuhar MJ, Yamamura HI: Light microscopic autoradiographic localization of cholinergic muscarinic sites in rat brain. *Proc Soc Neurosci* 1974;4:294.
16. Kuhar MJ, Yamamura HI: Light autoradiographic localization of cholinergic muscarinic receptors in rat brain by specific binding of a potent antagonist. *Nature* 1975;253:560–561.

17. Kuhar MJ, Yamamura HI: Localization of cholinergic muscarinic receptors in rat brain by light microscopic radioautography. *Brain Res* 1976; 110:229–243.
18. Uhl GR, Goodman RR, Kuhar MJ, et al: Immunohistochemical mapping of enkephalin-containing cell bodies, fibers and nerve terminals in the brainstem of the rat. *Brain Res* 1979;166:75–94.
19. Goldstein A, Cox BM: Opioid peptides (endorphins) in pituitary and brain. *Psychoneuroendocrinology* 1977;2:11–16.
20. Uhl GR, Childers SR, Snyder, SH: Opioid peptides and the opiate receptor in Ganong WF, Martini L (eds): *Frontiers in Neuroendocrinology.* New York, Raven Press, 1978, vol 5.
21. Terenius L: Endogenous peptides and analgesia. *Annu Rev Pharmacol Toxicol* 1978;18:189–204.
22. Hokfelt T, Ljungdahl A, Terenius L, et al: Immunohistochemical analysis of peptide pathways possibly related to pain and analgesia: Enkephalin and substance P. *Proc Natl Acad Sci USA* 1977;74:3081–3085.
23. Sar M, Stumpf WE: Immunohistochemical localization of enkephalin in rat brain and spinal cord. *J Comp Neurol* 1978;182:17–38.
24. Frederickson RCA: Enkephalin pentapeptides: A review of current evidence for a physiological role in vertebrate neurotransmission. *Life Sci* 1977;21:23–42.
25. Simantov R, Kuhar MJ, Pasternak GW, et al: The regional distribution of a morphine-like factor enkephalin in monkey brain. *Brain Res* 1976; 106:189–197.

18 Psychotropic Drugs and Chronic Pain

Gavril W. Pasternak

The management of patients with chronic pain is one of the most challenging problems in clinical medicine. Acute pain is usually easily controlled with a variety of drugs, especially the opiate narcotics, but chronic pain presents more difficult problems since the beneficial effects of opiates are diminished by the development of tolerance, the risk of addiction, and other side effects. Recently, a combination of psychotropic drugs, especially antidepressants and phenothiazines, have been reported to relieve some patients with chronic pain.[1-4] This chapter addresses the use and the possible pharmacological mechanisms of action of these drugs.

The Clinical Use of Psychotropic Drugs for Chronic Pain

That some phenothiazine drugs are analgesic has been known for a long time. In the 1950s, a number of investigators reported that several phenothiazine drugs potentiated the duration and intensity of opiate analgesia and even provided analgesic relief alone, although occasional reports were contradictory. These drugs were used extensively as preoperative medication in anesthesia and were generally found to be as good as the narcotics. Although several phenothiazines are effective analgesics, the most potent is methotrimeprazine. Methotrimeprazine had been extensively used in Europe and won acceptance in this country after a classic study by Lasagna and DeKornfeld.[5] These investigators compared methotrimeprazine and morphine in a double-blind protocol involving postoperative pain. The results indicated that methotrimeprazine (15 mg) provided analgesia equivalent to morphine (10 mg). Montilla et al[6] also found methotrimeprazine (15 mg) to be equianalgetic to morphine (10 mg) in patients with postoperative pain, herpes zoster, fractures, and pleurisy, although sedation appeared to be more pronounced with methotrimeprazine than morphine. Moore and Dundee[7] investigated the analgesic properties of several phenothiazines in an experimental pain model. Some phenothiazines were analgetic, but others were not. Although analgetic phenothiazines do not produce tolerance, addiction, or serious toxicity, high doses may be limited by postural hypotension, sedation and, on occasion, tardive dyskinesias.

Antidepressants have also been extensively used for pain control, especially in conjunction with phenothiazines. Most studies investigating the analgetic potency of antidepressants have been conducted in patients with chronic pain. One of the early studies investigated patients with refractory pain due to herpes zoster.[4] Using amitriptyline (40 to 100 mg/day), the authors reported good or complete relief of pain in 11 of 12 patients. They found that relief usually started in one to two weeks but only reached its maximal effects in four weeks. Additional reports by Taub and Collins[3] and Merskey and Hester[2] also suggested that antidepressants are of benefit in chronic pain. Unfortunately, these last two reports are not well controlled and also investigated the concurrent use of a phenothiazine.

Amitriptyline has been studied in patients with migraine.[1] The drug reduces the severity and frequency of the headaches and migraine-associated symptoms such as nausea, vomiting, visual problems, and even hemiparesis. The average time of therapy needed before obtaining beneficial results was about nine days. There appears to be only weak correlation between migraine and depression and no correlation between migraine improvement and depression improvement.[1] Although the results are not conclusive, they suggest that antidepressants may relieve pain specifically and not as a consequence to relieving depression.

Opiate Receptors and Enkephalins

Since the initial description of specific opiate receptors within mammalian brain,[8-10] our understanding of the mechanisms of opiate action has expanded dramatically. The opiate receptors are localized within the brain[11] in the same regions which are analgesic to the microinjection morphine.[12] The receptors are restricted to gray matter and their subcellular localization to pinched off nerve terminals or synaptosomes, suggesting that these receptors might be part of a new neurotransmitter system within the brain. The finding by Hughes et al[13] of an endogenous material from brain extracts with opiate-like actions in his bioassay system, substantiated by Terenius and Wahlstrom[14] and Pasternak et al[15] using receptor binding assay systems, furthered the transmitter concept. This material, enkephalin, was subsequently sequenced and named by Hughes et al.[16] As with the receptor, the enkephalins are localized to specific regions of brain associated opiate receptors[17] as well as to synaptosomes.[18] Thus, the enkephalins do appear to be a distinct neurotransmitter system within the brain.

The discovery of this system proved to be very important in understanding previous observations describing analgesia from electrical stimulation of brain which could be blocked by the very specific narcotic antagonist, naloxone.[19] This analgesia could be produced only by stimulating brain regions subsequently demonstrating high levels of enkephalins and endorphins. The combination of all these studies imply that the brain indeed does have a neurotransmitter system which, if activated, can produce analgesia.

Other studies have described another group of opiate-like peptides, the endorphins. Initially discovered by Goldstein's group,[20] these pituitary peptides are made from the same precursor protein as adrenocorticotropin hormone (ACTH). Unlike enkephalin, they appear to be hormones and are secreted into the blood stream by the same stimuli which release ACTH.

Neurotransmitter Interactions in Opiate and Stimulation Analgesia

The enkephalin system appears to be intimately related to pain mechanisms. It has already been demonstrated that release of enkephalin by electrical stimulation can produce opiate-like analgesia. A major question remaining in our understanding of clinical pain is the normal, physiological mechanism which releases the enkephalins. Neurons within the brain have very extensive and diverse inputs from other nerve cells. Modulation of enkephalin release will probably be mediated by a variety of additional neurotransmitters. In addition, the enkephalin neurons are probably only one link in a longer chain of neurons which finally produce clinical analgesia. Alteration of other neurotransmitters within the circuit might also alter pain perception.

The similarities between morphine and stimulation analgesia and that presumed due to the enkephalin systems suggest that studies on the interaction of established neurotransmitters with morphine and stimulation analgesia might prove useful in our understanding of pain perception. Although many putative neurotransmitters have been described recently, most work addressing the interaction of neurotransmitters and analgesia has focused on the catecholamines and serotonin. Many investigators have demonstrated a correlation between the general levels of monoamines in the central nervous system and the efficacy of morphine and stimulation analgesia. In general, pretreatment of animals with either reserpine or tetrabenazine to deplete amine levels prior to analgesia testing reduced the effectiveness of morphine and stimulation analgesia. If this were a specific effect, elevation of monoamines by administration of monoamine oxidase (MAO) inhibitors should potentiate analgesia. These expected findings were confirmed by several laboratories. These initial studies prompted many investigators to study individual monoamines more carefully (Tables 18-1 to 18-3).

Table 18-1
Neurotransmitters and Analgesia

Neurotransmitter	Morphine Analgesia	Stimulation Analgesia
Serotonin	increase	increase
Dopamine	increase	increase
Norepinephrine		
Alpha receptor actions	decrease	decrease
Beta receptor actions	no effect	no effect

Numerous techniques were used to investigate serotonin function in the brain. These have included the direct administration of serotonin into the brain as well as manipulating serotonin levels by pharmacological and physical means. The most direct method, injection of serotonin into the cerebral ventricle, potentiates morphine analgesia.[21] In addition, intraventricular serotonin reversed the effects of reserpine on morphine action described earlier, strengthening previous observations that serotonin precursors like tryptophan and 5-hydroxytryptophan enhance morphine's actions. Serotonin has similar effects on stimulation analgesia.[22,23] As with morphine analgesia, decreased stimulation analgesia from a generalized depletion of monoamines by tetrabenazine can be reversed by administration of serotonin precursors. Most of the serotonin neurons within the brain are localized to the dorsal raphe nuclei in the brainstem. Early work on this neurotransmitter established that stimulation of this region increased the release of serotonin, while ablation of the area markedly decreased the amount of serotonin within the brain. In a series of papers, Samanin et al[24,25] demonstrated that stimulation of the dorsal raphe nuclei, but not the lateral dorsal raphe nuclei (which has little serotonin), markedly heightened morphine's peak antinociceptive effect and its duration of action. In complementary experiments, they report that destruction of the dorsal raphe nuclei depleted brain serotonin almost 80% and decreased morphine's analgesic potency. Pharmacological blockade of serotonin synthesis by p-chlorophenylalanine also depletes serotonin in the brain with a corresponding decrease in morphine and stimulation analgesia. These results clearly show that the serotonin system is an important link in the generalized expression of analgesia.

Table 18-2
Neurotransmitter Effects on Morphine Analgesia

	Morphine Analgesia
Monoamines	
Enhancement: MAO inhibitors	increase
Depletion:	
Tetrabenazine	decrease
Reserpine	decrease
Reserpine + L-DOPA	analgesia restored
Serotonin	
Enhancement:	
5-hydroxytryptophan	increase
Stimulation raphe nuclei	increase
Intraventricular serotonin	increase
Depletion:	
P-chlorophenylalanine	decrease
Lesions of raphe nuclei	decrease
Catecholamines	
Depletion: α-Methyltyrosine	decrease
Enhancement: L-DOPA	increase
Norepinephrine	
Intraventricular NE	decrease
Dopamine-β-hydroxylase inhibitors	
Diethyldithiocarbamate	increase
1-phenyl-3(2-thiazolyl)-2-thiourea	increase
Alpha receptor agonist: clonidine	decrease
Alpha receptor blockers:	
Phentolamine	increase
Phenoxybenzamine	increase
Beta receptor blockers:	
Propranolol	no effect
Practolol	no effect

Because of common synthetic pathways, the catecholamines are more difficult to study. The pathway starts at tyrosine, proceeds to dopamine, and then to norepinephrine via the enzyme dopamine-β-hydroxylase. Interference in the synthesis of dopamine, therefore, also affects norepinephrine. α-Methyltyrosine blocks the synthesis of both dopamine and norepinephrine and lowers their concentration within the brain. Animals pretreated with this drug display a marked reduction in both morphine and stimulation analgesia. L-DOPA, a catecholamine precursor which bypasses this enzymatic block, repletes dopamine and norepinephrine levels and restores both types of analgesia. Unfortunately, these studies do not discriminate between dopamine and norepinephrine effects. When norepinephrine was infused directly into the cerebral ventricles, morphine analgesia was depressed.[21] Pharmacologically depleting only norepinephrine levels with dopamine-β-hydroxylase inhibitors which block the conversion of dopamine to norepinephrine enhances both morphine and stimulation analgesia. However, depletion of both dopamine and norepinephrine by reserpine or α-methyltyrosine have an opposite effect. These results might be explained if dopamine enhances analgesia while norepinephrine inhibits it. Treatments and drugs which affect both drugs might yield mixed results, depending upon the relative effects on the two transmitters.

Analysis of norepinephrine's effects on analgesia are also complicated by its two types of receptors and their pharmacological effects, alpha and beta. Clonidine, a norepinephrine-like drug which acts at the alpha receptor, depresses morphine analgesia.[26] Specific alpha receptor blockers such as phentolamine and phenoxybenzamine increase morphine analgesia, and there are reports that alpha receptors can even pro-

Table 18-3
Neurotransmitter Effects on Stimulation Analgesia

	Stimulation Analgesia
Monoamines	
Depletion:	
Tetrabenazine	decrease
Tetrabenazine + L-DOPA	analgesia restored
Tetrabenazine + 5-hydroxytryptophan	analgesia restored
Catecholamines	
Enhancement:	
L-DOPA	small increase
Depletion:	
α-Methyltyrosine	decrease
α-Methyltyrosine + L-DOPA	analgesia restored
Depletion of NE	
Disulfiram	increase
Serotonin	
Depletion:	
P-chlorphenylalanine	decrease

duce analgesia without morphine.[26] Drugs specific for beta receptors are without effect.

Pain perception seems to be mediated by a variety of neurotransmitter systems (Table 18-1). Both serotonin and dopamine appear to be important in the production of analgesia while norepinephrine antagonizes it through its alpha adrenergic system. Alteration of any of these three systems can have dramatic effects on pain sensation. These investigations still present problems with a molecular analysis of analgesic mechanisms. The results do not tell us whether these transmitters a) act upon the enkephalin system directly, b) parallel the enkephalin system and end on a final common pathway, or c) act further along the circuits from the enkephalin neurons. In fact, these systems might actually work upon other transmitters which in turn affect the pain perception:

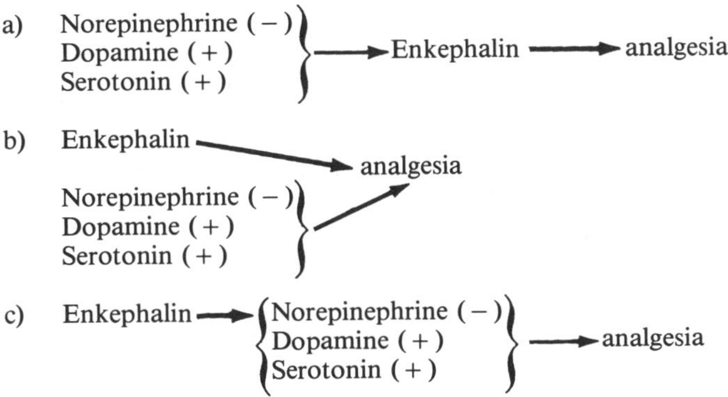

Psychotropic Drugs and Pain

The analgesic usefulness of psychotropic drugs appears to be well established. While their pharmacological mechanisms of action remain obscure, they are known to have numerous actions on central nervous system monoamines. It is interesting to speculate about analgesic mechanisms, using some of the data on monoaminergic transmitter systems presented earlier.

Pharmacologically, the phenothiazines are proposed to exert their antischizophrenic actions through blockade of the dopamine receptor.[27] The blockade of dopamine receptors by neuroleptics might be expected to decrease analgesia, but some neuroleptic drugs bind to other types of receptors. Different phenothiazines, butyrophenones, and thioxanthenes have also been noted to differ markedly in their side-effects when given at equi-antischizophrenic doses. Peroutka et al[28] have examined the molecular binding of these neuroleptics and have found that their affinity for other neurotransmitter receptors may be the same or higher than their affinity for the dopamine receptor. They have proposed that interaction with cholinergic receptors might explain why certain phenothiazines have a lower incidence of parkinsonian-like symptoms. Likewise, certain neuroleptics have an affinity for alpha norepinephrine receptors which is higher than the classical alpha blockers phenoxybenzamine and phentolamine. Alpha receptor blockade, which potentiates morphine and stimulation analgesia, might explain their analgesic actions.

Another possible mechanism of analgesic action of psychotropic drugs might be explained by findings from Hong et al.[29] When rats were treated chronically with a variety of neuroleptics, the concentrations of methionine-enkephalin within the brain was markedly increased. The ability to elevate enkephalin levels varied between the neuroleptics, with haloperidol doubling the amount of enkephalin and pimazide and chlorpromazine producing only a 40% to 50% increase. The increase in enkephalins was dose dependent and also time dependent, taking approximately three weeks for maximal effect. This increase in brain enkephalins might be important in decreasing pain sensation.

Antidepressants also produce profound effects on central nervous system amines. These drugs have been found to inhibit the presynaptic uptake of the catecholamines and serotonin, potentiating their action.[30] Certain drugs, such as amitriptyline and imipramine, have greater effects on serotonin reuptake while others, such as desipramine and nortriptyline, are more potent on norepinephrine reuptake. Potentiation of the serotonergic system by amitriptyline might be expected to potentiate analgesic systems in the central nervous system. Recent reports[31] have also suggested that long-term treatment with antidepressants decreases the sensitivity of alpha norepinephrine receptors. Since alpha norepinephrine effects antagonize the analgesic systems, a depression of alpha receptor sensitivity might decrease painful sensations. Interestingly, the necessity of several weeks of treatment to obtain the decrease in receptor sensitivity corresponds very well to the time interval needed for clinical effectiveness.

Conclusions

The clinical use of psychotropic drugs for pain is increasing. Although definitive studies are lacking, the bulk of evidence currently available suggests they are efficacious. The presence of an enkephalinergic analgesic system within the brain helps explain some basic mechanisms of analgesia, and the interaction of various neurotransmitters on this analgetic system has proposed somc hypotheses of psychotropic drug action. These potential mechanisms of action remain highly speculative and will probably prove too simplistic.

However, they provide a possible hypothesis of the molecular basis of analgesia from psychotropic drugs and can be used to design further studies in pain perception.

REFERENCES

1. Couch JR, Ziergler DK, Hassanein R: Amitriptyline on the prophylaxis of migraine. *Neurology* 1976;26:121–127.
2. Merskey H, Hester RA: The treatment of chronic pain with psychotropic drugs. *Postgrad Med J* 1972;48:594–598.
3. Taub A, Collins WF: Observations on the treatment of denervation dysesthesia with psychotropic drugs: Postherpetic neuralgia, anesthesia dolorosa, peripheral neuropathy, in, Bonica JJ (ed): *Advances in Neurology*. New York, Raven Press, vol 4, 1974, pp 309–315.
4. Woodeforde JM, Dwyer B, McEwen BW, et al: Treatment of postherpetic neuralgia. *Med J Aust* 1965;2:869–872.
5. Lasagna L, DeKornfeld JJ: Methotrimeprazine: A new phenothiazine derivative with analgetic properties. *JAMA* 1961;178:887–890.
6. Montilla E, Frederick W, Cass L: Analgesic effect of methotrinephrazine and morphine. *Arch Intern Med* 1963;111:725–728.
7. Moore JA, Dundee JW: Alterations to somatic pain associated with anesthesia. VII The effects of nine phenothiazine derivatives. *Br J Anaesth* 1961;33:422–431.
8. Pert CB, Snyder SH: Opiate receptor: Demonstration in nervous tissue. *Science* 1973;179:1011–1014.
9. Simon EJ, Hiller JM, Delman I: Stereospecific binding of the potent narcotic analgesic ^{3}H-etorphine to rat brain homoginate. *Proc Natl Acad Sci USA* 1973;70:1947–1949.
10. Terenius L: Characteristics of the "receptor" for narcotic analgesics in synaptic plasma membrane fraction from rat brain. *Acta Pharmacol Toxicol* 1973;32:377–384.
11. Kuhar M, Pert CB, Snyder SH: Regional distribution of opiate receptor binding in monkey and human brain. *Nature* 1973;245:447–450.
12. Pert A, Yaksh T: Sites of morphine-induced analgesia in the primate brain: Relation to pain pathways. *Brain Res* 1974;80:135–140.
13. Hughes J: Isolation of an endogenous compound from the brain with pharmacological properties similar to morphine. *Brain Res* 1975;88:295–308.
14. Terenius L, Wahlstrom A: Morphine-like ligand for opiate receptors in human CSF. *Life Sci* 1975;16:1759–1764.
15. Pasternak GW, Goodman R, Snyder SH: An endogenous morphine-like factor in mammalian brain. *Life Sci* 1975;16:1765–1769.
16. Hughes J, Smith TW, Kosterlitz HW, et al: Identification of two related pentapeptides from the brain with potent opiate agonist activity. *Nature* 1975;258:577–579.
17. Simantov R, Kuhar MJ, Pasternak GW, et al: The regional distribution of a morphine-like factor enkephalin in monkey brain. *Brain Res* 1976; 106:189–197.
18. Simantov R, Snowman AM, Snyder SH: A morphine-like factor "enkephalin" in rat brain: Subcellular localization. *Brain Res* 1976; 107:650–657.

19. Mayer DJ, Wolfe TL, Akil H, et al: Analgesia from electrical stimulation in the brainstem of the rat. *Science* 1971;174:1351–1354.
20. Cox BM, Opheim KE, Teschemacher H, et al: A peptide-like substance from pituitary that acts like morphine. *Life Sci* 1975;16:1777–1782.
21. Sparkes CG, Spencer PSJ: Antinociceptive activity of morphine after injection of biogenic amines in the cerebral ventricles of the conscious rat. *Br J Pharmacol* 1971;42:230–241.
22. Akil H, Liebeskind JC: Monoaminergic mechanisms of stimulation-produced analgesia. *Brain Res* 1975;94:279–296.
23. Akil H, Mayer D: Antagonism of stimulation-produced analgesia by p-CPA, a serotonin synthesis inhibitor. *Brain Res* 1972;44:692–696.
24. Samanin R, Gumulka E, Valzelli L: Reduced effect of morphine in midbrain raphe lesioned rats. *Eur J Pharmacol* 1970;10:339–343.
25. Samanin R, Valzelli L: Increase of morphine induced analgesia by stimulation of the nucleus raphe dorsalis. *Eur J Pharmacol* 1971;16:298–302.
26. Cicero TJ, Meyer ER, Smithhoff BR: Alpha adrenergic blocking agents: Antinociceptive activity and enhancement of morphine-induced analgesia. *J Pharmacol Exp Ther* 1974;189:72–82.
27. Burt DR, Creese L, Snyder SH: Properties of ^{3}H-haloperidol and ^{3}H-dopamine binding associated with dopamine receptors in calf brain membranes. *Mol Pharmacol* 1976;12:800–812.
28. Peroutka SS, U'Prichard DC, Greenberg DA, et al: Neuroleptic drug interactors with norepinephrine alpha receptor binding sites in rat brain. *Neuropharmacology* 1977;16:549–556.
29. Hong JS, Yang HY, Fratta W, et al: Rat striatal methionine-enkephalin content after chronic treatment with cataleptogenic and noncataleptogenic antischizophrenic drugs. *J Pharmacol Exp Ther* 1978;205:141–147.
30. Sulser F, Sanders-Bush E: Effects of drugs on amines in the CNS. *Ann Rev Pharmacol* 1971;11:209.
31. Crews FT, Smith CB: Presynaptic alpha-receptor subsensitivity after long-term antidepressant treatment. *Science* 1978;202:322–324.

19 The Clinical Management of Chronic Pain

Richard G. Black

The constellation of syndromes characterizing the patient with a chronic intractable pain complaint is characteristic enough to constitute a disease entity we shall call the chronic pain syndrome.[1] Regardless of the duration, its presence is confirmed by a significant alteration in the patient's life style, his relations with other individuals, and a failure to show any progressive improvement, while at the same time rarely becoming worse. In fact, the condition of the patient with the chronic pain syndrome is extremely stable. They become neither better nor worse for many years while continuing to seek help from the health care system and submitting to its therapies. The victim of the chronic pain syndrome suffers from intractable, often multiple pain complaints, many of which are inappropriate to existing physical problems or illnesses. There is a history of multiple physician contacts and many nonproductive diagnostic procedures. There is excessive preoccupation with the complaints both on the part of the patient, and family and friends as well. All sufferers of the chronic pain syndrome have an audience for their suffering and, in a most skilled manner, play to that audience to obtain their immediate gains. Features of depression, anxiety, and neuroticism are present.[1,2] The victim of this syndrome has no realistic plans for the future nor patience with any therapy requiring time or active participation on his part.

The chronic pain syndrome is, in its later stages, accompanied by excessive use of short-acting medications, particularly analgesics, but also benzodiazepines and hypnotics. It is the chronic long-term use of such medications that produces a mild toxic or metabolic organic brain syndrome which further confuses the diagnostic picture and makes it impossible for the victim of this disease to recover by himself without long-term support.[3,4] Patients with such a problem often present themselves in such a strong manner, with support from family and friends, that surgery or further prescriptions for these same drugs may seem appropriate to the unwary physician.

Disabling secondary problems soon follow the establishment of the chronic pain syndrome. Anxiety and depression develop from chronic pain which, by its very presence, leads its victim to despair at the seemingly useless and endless nature of his suffering. Concern over loss of income and work, and the patient's own failing mental and physical abilities, serve to increase anxiety. These same factors add to the depression that was already present as part of the syndrome. The use of narcotic and synthetic analgesics, as well as the benzodiazepines, not only can cause depression but serve to magnify any depression present.[5] Sleep patterns become altered either through the presence of nociception or through the use of short-acting analgesics on a prn basis. Even the use of hypnotics on a regular basis serve to disrupt the percentage of sleep time spent in each of the various components making up the regular physiological sleep pattern. This results in an abnormal and unrestful sleep period which, on a regular basis, significantly decreases the feeling of well-being. Soon, this primary disturbance of the circadian rhythm has established itself, and progressive physical and mental deterioration follow.

Since pain is an acceptable affliction in our society, and one especially worthy of sympathy, environmental rewards in the guise of attention by well-meaning friends and family act to sustain the individual continuing in his role as the patient or ill person.[6,7] This acts to increase illness behavior and puts the individual in the difficult position of, once having the special benefits of being ill, not being able to justify acting well again. In addition, many activities that might make the individual feel a worthwhile and functional member of his family or society are taken away by well-meaning friends who end up unintentionally increasing the duration and severity of the chronic pain syndrome. Careful examination of the situation from a behavioral viewpoint shows that both patient and family must make difficult, sometimes impossible, changes to break out of the vicious self-propagating circle of illness behavior. They must decrease, modify, or stop altogether some behaviors or actions they have been doing that gave an immediate reward or enjoyment, and they must start to do some new things, often difficult and undesired, for which the negative consequences of failure to perform are remote and not previously experienced.[8]

The chronic pain patient in his sometimes desperate search for help is also exposed to a high risk of iatrogenic complications at the hands of well-meaning physicians. These physicians are not malicious, but are practicing according to the experience gained during their years of training. If the patient with a chronic pain syndrome seeks out the assistance of a surgeon in solving his pain problem, he may expect surgery in return since this is the therapy the surgeon deals in and is paid for doing. The surgical approach in this type of patient at first consists of diagnostic or corrective surgery such as laparotomy, laminectomy, hysterectomy, or discectomy. Later, when relief of pain has not been obtained, more surgery may be done, this time directly on the nervous system to cut pain pathways, implant stimulators, or alter behavior. It is indeed a tribute to the organization of the human nervous system that it is able to successfully negate all of these attempts at pain relief within six months to several years, and a comment on the surgical ethic that many patients with a chronic pain syndrome have undergone 10 to 20 surgical procedures, and some even 40 or more! This situation, it should be emphasized, does not imply that surgeons are malicious or too ready to operate, but with their training and limited skills on one hand, and the pressure of a patient and his family demanding help on the other, it is sometimes difficult to refuse an operation that is known from experience to work very well so many times in so many cases, but all on acute pain problems. An added incentive for surgery is the readiness of third party carriers to pay for recognized procedures and their reluctance to finance alternative therapies such as biofeedback, group psychology, and rehabilitation.

Abuse of short-acting analgesic medications is the primary factor responsible for sustaining the chronic pain syndrome in a majority of patients. These patients and their families have come to believe that a simple taking of a pill will in some miraculous way solve all of their problems. The billion dollar annual market in over-the-counter analgesic drugs illustrates this problem. Many physicians who have been taught the proper use of analgesics for acute pain and who, through experience, have confirmed their efficacy in this area apply the same therapeutic regimes to patients with chronic pain and ultimately make the patient much worse. Unfortunately, the long-term use of short-acting analgesics on a prn basis results in escalation of their use, depression of the activity of neurotransmitters, and a resulting increase in the intensity of pain as reported by the patient. Nonanalgesic drugs, such as the tranquilizers, hypnotics, and muscle relaxants, also have cumulative toxic side effects and play as important a role in this problem as do the analgesics. Confusion of higher thought processes, similar to an organic brain syndrome, which results from continued use of prescription and over-the-counter drugs, is ignored by many examining physicians even though it may contribute significantly to misdiagnosis and inappropriate therapy. Chronic users of short-acting analgesic medications report less pain after these medications are discontinued.[2,4] So important, and sometimes subtle or even occult, is this problem that a basic principle in the management of pain patients is that whenever excessive or chronic use of medication is even suspected, it must be withdrawn before a meaningful diagnostic evaluation can be attempted.

Another way of viewing the problem of patients suffering from the chronic pain syndrome is to consider them as failures of an efficient health care delivery system. These individuals represent a relatively small percentage of patients who consume a relatively large percentage of the health care services. The system with which they interface is designed to increase both the physicians' efficiency and use of facilities to permit more patients to be treated in less time at a lower cost. Unfortunately, inherent in this plan is a reduction of physician-patient contact time. A certain percentage of patients, those with more obscure problems, such as multisystem disease, psychological overlay, or dependency needs, do not respond to this type of approach and begin seeing other physicians. This help-seeking behavior becomes more desperate and yet more stereotyped and nonproductive. Direct access to specialists is easily obtained with the resulting management becoming more and more technical as the elusive psychological and sociological factors comprising the art of medicine are ignored. Unfortunately, these patients require, even demand, a greater expenditure of time than the average patient, and many physicians are understandably reluctant to spend the required time with these patients. It is obvious that more of the same, whether it be brief physician contact, medications, or surgery, is not going to help, and that a new and different approach, such as offered by a pain clinic or pain treatment center or sensitive physician skilled in the management of chronic pain, is needed.[2,9,10]

Organization of a Chronic Pain Treatment Center

There are over 450 chronic pain treatment centers in the United States today. Of this number, only 20 are what one may consider multidisciplinary. One is faced with many considerations when organizing a chronic pain treatment center, but first and foremost is the purpose of such a center.

The aims of all centers do not overlap. Some treatment facilities seek only to provide pain relief. Others are designed to merely modify the response to the pain, thereby altering behavior. Therefore, the purpose of the center determines the organization of it.

At a minimum, there are seven areas where a clinician may intervene. Of paramount importance is the need to diagnose the etiology of the chronic pain complaint. While at first this seems obvious, there are in fact pain treatment centers that make no efforts in this direction. This is a serious oversight, since a large component of a patient's perception of pain is fear, ie, "What is it that is causing my pain, since pain means something is wrong?" The diagnostic approach is best conducted in an inpatient multidisciplinary center. Outpatient centers and/or unimodal centers that employ only one treatment technique do not lend themselves to fulfilling the role of a diagnostic center.

Once diagnosis has been established, a treatment center should function as an educational experience for the patient. Didactic classes on appropriate drug use, proper exercise, and, most importantly, an explanation to the patient of the anatomy and physiology of their specific pain problem will provide a reduction of any fear associated with the pain itself. It also will improve compliance with the chronic pain treatment center program.

After diagnosis and education are initiated, alteration of the patient's medication is critical. For a host of reasons, mentioned elsewhere in this chapter and by other authors in this volume, it is imperative to eliminate the use of all narcotics, hypnotics, sedatives, and benzodiazepine tranquilizers. The rationale for this approach is quite simple. Whatever benefit a patient derives from the use of the medications listed above is either far outweighed by the harmful side effects, or an equally effective but less harmful medication is available. The best way to control medication is in a residential setting.

The fourth area of concern in a chronic pain treatment center is the diagnosis and treatment of depression and anxiety that either antedated the pain or, much more likely, arose as a result of the pain, as discussed in Chapter 1. The literature is replete with articles which indicate that the perception of pain is worsened by anxiety and depression, and the patients themselves feel that these emotional factors create as many problems for them as the pain itself.

The fifth area of concern is directed toward making the chronic pain patient more functional. This may be accomplished by a variety of means, ranging from behavior modification to exercise classes. If one is committed to a behavioral approach, then this is best accomplished with an inpatient unit. However, if one merely relies on exercise, then any supervised group setting could be effective. In fact, vocational rehabilitation programs may be best accomplished using on-site training of individuals, which obviously does not take place in a formalized treatment center.

The sixth, and one of the most critical, area is improved family relationships. Family counseling can be accomplished in either an inpatient or outpatient setting, but one may find that an inpatient setting lends itself to this form of therapy far better than an outpatient treatment center. The major factor is the removal of the individual with chronic pain from the home environment. This alteration in the family dynamics permits a degree of objectivity and reflection for both the chronic pain patient and his family, that otherwise might not occur if the patient remained in his usual environment.

The final aim of a chronic pain treatment center is, of course, pain relief. Of course, if the pain problem is amenable to the type of therapy offered, then any unimodal center can be effective, on either an outpatient or inpatient basis; eg, a sympathetic dystrophy, once properly diagnosed, can be treated by repetitive sympathetic blocks. However, if the treatment fails to produce pain relief, one is then faced with a disappointed individual who needs other modalities of therapy to help him cope with the pain he will have the rest of his life, and to improve his level of functioning. For this reason, one cannot consider a facility that merely attempts to remove pain as a true pain treatment center.

If one accepts the above-mentioned seven purposes of a pain treatment center (diagnosis, education, medication regulation, treatment of anxiety and depression, improved level of functioning for the patient, improved family relationship, and pain relief) as desirable goals, then the next question should be "How do I effect these goals?" The two variables to consider are the choice of a unimodal vs multidisciplinary approach, and whether or not to conduct therapy on an inpatient or outpatient basis.

The pros and cons of unimodal treatment (block centers, transcutaneous nerve stimulator centers, hypnosis centers, etc), when compared to a multidisciplinary center, are quite obvious. A unimodal center can offer a specialized form of treatment at which the practitioners at the clinic are highly skilled. They, therefore, can quickly 1) determine if the treatment is appropriate for a patient, and 2) skillfully administer the treatment. However, they do not have extensive diagnostic capabilities that allow them to determine what is wrong with a patient who is not suitable for their treatment, and do not have the ability to support a patient if he is 1) not suitable for their particular type of treatment, or 2) if their type of treatment fails. In counterdistinction, a multidisciplinary center has increased diagnostic capabilities and can provide many treatment programs that allow a clinician the choice of selecting the one(s) best suited for his patient. Therefore, a patient is better served at a multidisciplinary pain treatment center.

The other consideration of treatment pertains to the use of an inpatient vs outpatient setting. Obviously, an outpatient setting will have less cost, and fewer personnel. However, in an outpatient environment, the clinician loses control over a number of factors, of which there are three notable examples. First, and foremost, is the inability to control and monitor drug intake, especially narcotic, hypnotic, and tranquilizing drugs. Even on inpatient units, patients smuggle in drugs; so one may surely surmise that, on an outpatient basis, there is no certain way a physician may exert any control over drug intake. As a corollary to that, one cannot observe and, therefore, modify patient behavior. This element of "pain control" is the cornerstone of a great many treatment programs, and is virtually impossible to manage on an outpatient basis. This is due, in large part, to the role the family plays in maintaining chronic pain behavior on the part of the patient. Only in an inpatient setting can family influences be modified and controlled. Therefore, it is the opinion of this author, shared by many who treat chronic pain patients, that the most efficient modality of treatment is a multidisciplinary inpatient chronic pain treatment center.

Pain as a Complaint

Pain is the most common reason for a patient to consult a health care professional or even an individual offering services peripheral to what might be considered recognized and proper care. Yet, this complaint of pain often remains poorly understood and frequently mismanaged. The work pain may have many meanings from an annoyance, such as a pain in the neck to expressing extreme nociception as with an abscessed tooth or broken bone.[11] The words may be the same, the sensation invisible, and the display of suffering unrelated to the intensity of the nociceptive sensation. Human suffering expressed as pain with hidden meanings of depression, anxiety, fear, or even an untenable social situation, is too often accepted by the health care professional, relatives, and friends as meaning the patient has a medically or surgically correctable illness.

Attempts to define the meaning of the word pain range from C.S. Lewis's[12] statement, "Pain is an experience whether physical or mental which the patient dislikes," to R.A. Sternbach's[13] relativistic definition, "Pain is an abstract concept which an observer may use to describe a personal, private sense of hurt, a harmful stimulus which signals current or impending tissue damage, and a pattern of responses which operate to protect the organism from harm." An acceptable working definition of pain is "an unpleasant experience which we primarily associate with tissue damage or describe in terms of tissue damage or both."[14] This proposal of Merskey combines subjective experience, an apparent physical pain generator, and the response by which an outside observer would agree one was in pain. Melzack and Torgerson[15] have suggested that pain might be described in terms of several sensory and affective dimensions and have made a substantial contribution concerning the language used to describe pain.

Physicians wonder why certain patients have not responded to or do not continue to respond to surgical or medical interventions that have already been proven to be successful forms of therapy. These very patients are often blamed for their bad response to good therapy. When reevaluated with an approach that considers their complaint of pain as an expression of suffering, and with an attempt to find the cause of the suffering in a comprehensive manner, it becomes apparent that inappropriate and even harmful therapy has been done by early, sometimes routine, surgical or medical intervention. A new approach is required for this type of patient in order to avoid this problem. Even more important criteria must be found to identify these patients early in the course of their health care. Any approach to a patient with a chronic complaint of pain should consider the suffering of the patient to have components related to nociception, anxiety, depression, and a complex reaction to social, psychological, and environmental stresses.[1]

There is a recently acknowledged and significant difference between acute pain and chronic pain.[4,10] These are two distinctly different diseases having in common only the complaint of pain. The experiences of both physicians and patients with acute pain may be carried over into areas of chronic pain with disastrous results. The patient with minimal physical findings who complains of long-standing low back pain, vague abdominal discomfort, and myofascial problems may be treated in the same manner as a patient with an acute pain problem related to significant pathology. The usual drugs and surgery known to be successful for the acute problem are applied and only transiently help the patient who now becomes worse. Both the patient and physician become desperate, seeking stronger medications and more mutilating surgery, until each regards the other as being incompetent or psychologically disturbed. Referral is made to other specialists who have a try, until the patient becomes firmly labeled with the regrettable terms of "crock" and "crazy."

The highly specialized nature of the physician's training narrows his view of the patient's problem, and often eliminates all consideration except physical disease, biochemical disorders or extreme psychological problems. In the specialist, this tunnel vision may become even more extreme, being directed at one particular organ system or approach. The intense specialization of our medical training system and the lack of opportunity for residents in training to experience the long-term effects of their therapies before rotating to another service, contribute heavily to the lack of insight most specialists have toward other factors related to the patient's complaints and the long-term outcome of their own therapies.

To understand the meaning of a patient's complaint, attention must be directed to all of the components of his pain problem and the nature of chronic pain and its vast differences from acute pain must be appreciated.[1] Many definitions for chronic pain have been attempted that involve some element of time, generally six months.[4] The most significant factors differing chronic pain from acute pain are not time, but that the pain is no longer serving as a protective or warning signal and has become an end unto itself, and that the victim's lifestyle has been significantly changed by the disease. Chronic nociception must not be confused with the syndrome of chronic pain. There are many sufferers of arthritis who have chronic nociception but, in no way, can they be compared with the depressed dependent victims of chronic pain with their high incidence of medication dependency and disturbed psychosocial functioning.

A Recommended Diagnostic Approach to the Patient with Chronic Pain

The management of the unfortunate victim of chronic intractable pain depends for success on a correct diagnosis. Unless a correct diagnosis is made, inappropriate therapy will be done, but a correct diagnosis will lead to appropriate therapy. It is the meaning of diagnosis that is important in this statement, and especially important when dealing with the patient suffering from the chronic pain syndrome. A diagnosis must include all of the factors affecting the suffering of the patient. This includes his physical, psychological, sociological, and economic problems, most of which will be overlooked the more definite the diagnosis the patient presents with and the more specialized the training of his physician. A correct diagnosis is particularly difficult in patients with a chronic pain syndrome, since these individuals often come with an established diagnosis or label which may, on critical examination, be so inappropriate or outdated as to be dangerously useless. Often, this label is a mere description of a disease which may have little or no relation to the patient's pain problem, or else a pre-existing problem such as disc disease used to explain the pain from a myofascial problem or hamstring contractures.

By the time the patient has acquired the chronic pain syndrome, he has, by definition, failed the therapy offered by an efficient conventional health care system. A new approach is necessary. This may be received at a multidisciplinary pain treatment center, or even at the hands of an interested individual physician who is willing to take adequate time to make a systematic evaluation of the total problem.

In the conventional approach at first physical and, only later, possibly in desperation, psychological factors are evaluated. Sociological and economic factors are almost never considered except where compensation may be evoked to explain why a patient does not get better or litigation used as an excuse to avoid seeing a patient at all. In contrast, the patient with the chronic pain syndrome must be assessed simultaneously for all of these factors, physical, mental, and environmental.[1] It is essential that both the patient and the physician understand that these factors interrelate, and the patient's cooperation in the evaluation and his participation in his own care is essential. Participation of the spouse and other involved family members is also necessary, since the home situation may be the determining factor in maintaining the syndrome. Patients, and patients with a family who will not readily agree to such total management, will probably not improve with treatment and should be advised to return for help only when prepared to cooperate in their own care.

A diagnostic approach that has proven most useful with chronic pain patients involves fractionation of the patient's complaint into various components which are individually evaluated.[1] These components are then combined to form a pain profile for that individual patient at that particular time (Figure 19-1). The highest peaks in this profile are considered the major problem areas and are treated first in the course of the patient's management. This will bring about the greatest improvement in the chronic pain syndrome in the shortest time.

The components found most useful are as follows:

Somatogenic	This refers to the physical hurt or nociceptive component of the pain problem. It is divided into an acute component and a chronic component.
Anxiety	This refers to the patient's psychological state at the time of diagnosis. It is divided into state anxiety and trait anxiety.
Depression	This refers to the patient's degree of depression at the time of diagnosis. It is divided into endogenous depression, reactive depression, and depression secondary to use of medications, an exogenous chemical depression.

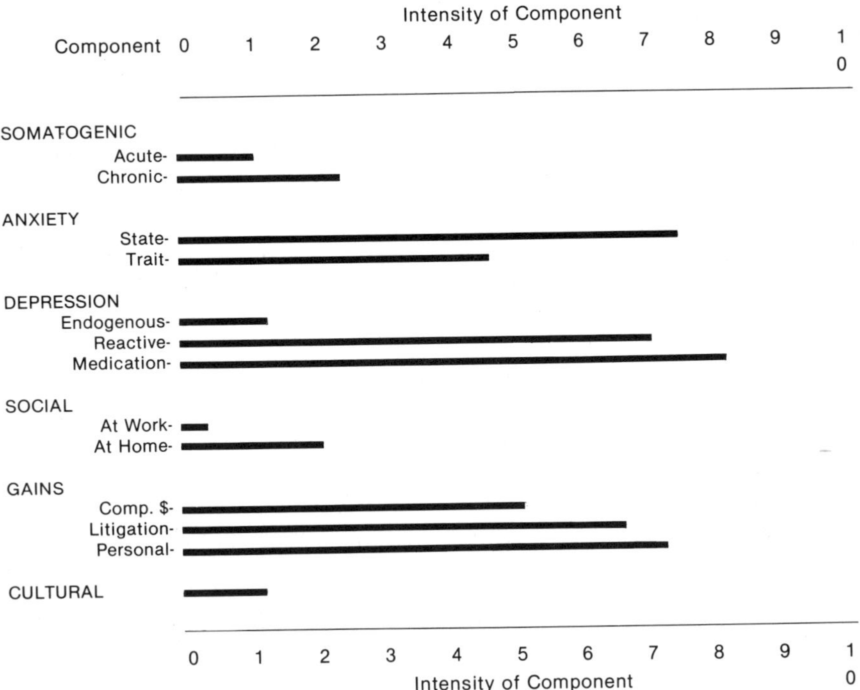

Figure 19-1 This reconstruction of a computer-generated graph demonstrates the magnitude of each of the components of suffering in the patient with a complaint of long-term chronic pain as described in the text. It is used therapeutically to direct treatment at those factors contributing most to the patient's "dis-ease." In this example, treatment of the nociceptive or somatic component alone with analgesics or surgery would make little difference to the patient's overall suffering.

Social	This factor refers to the stress present in the patient's social situation. It is divided into problems at work and problems at home.
Gains	This factor refers to gains received by the patient from his pain behavior. It is divided into gains from financial compensation, gains hoped for from litigation, and personal gains from family and friends.
Cultural	This refers to modifying factors peculiar to the individual patient's culture.

The usefulness of this approach is that once the physician is aware of the various components described, his attention is drawn to any problems in these areas. It will then be possible with directed questioning, simple psychological testing, the assistance of a social worker, and interviews with influential family members, to estimate a reasonably correct profile for the patient. Therapy may then be directed where it will be most effective and least harmful.

Recently, Dr Thomas Staats has developed a self-administered test that takes only 15 minutes of instruction time by the clinician. The test consists of a variety of well-known clinical tests, designed to measure three areas of a patient's life that influence his response to chronic pain and his perception of pain's impact on his life. These are 1) psychological traits of the individual, measured by the short form of the MMPI (Minnesota Multiphasic Personality Inventory), the A-type behavior rating scale, and the SCL-90 (Symptom Check List designed by Derogatis to measure the psychological state of the individual); 2) environmental factors that influence pain perception, as measured by the Holmes-Rahe Test of Recent Life Events and Life Stress; and 3) a physical scale designed to determine the impact of physical illness on the patient's life, as measured by the Hendler Screening Test for Chronic Back Pain Patients, and a physical/medical history. This test gives a three-dimensional rating of a patient, and is computer scored, so that the answers to the 466 questions are graphically displayed, and a single paragraph interpretation is offered for each of the three areas of evaluation: 1) psychological factors, 2) environmental factors, and 3) physical factors. Additional information about the test is available from Thomas Staats, PhD, Medicomp Corporation, 845 Margaret Place, Shreveport, Louisiana, 71101.

In summary, the diagnosis and treatment of chronic pain requires a multidisciplinary approach, and a multifactorial analysis of the various spheres of impact on a patient's life. Despite great advances within various branches of medicine, the analysis of chronic pain has defied almost all single approaches when applied without due consideration for the multifaceted nature of this disorder.

Management of Cancer Pain

Since the pain accompanying malignancies is often chronic in nature, requiring ongoing management over an extended period of time, a brief discussion of the use and effects of narcotics will be included here.

Kanner and Foley[16] have dealt with the issue of narcotics in cancer patients in a most comprehensive fashion. They feel that physicians *underuse* narcotics in medically ill patients, since most clinicians do not make the distinction between physical dependence and addiction. The authors feel that these two terms are not mutually inclusive, and further clarify the issue by offering several definitions. *Tolerance,* as defined by the World Health Organization, is a state in which an individual is less susceptible to the effect of a drug as the result of prior administration. *Physical dependence* is present when an abstinence syndrome appears, upon withdrawal of the drug. *Substance abuse* is defined as the use of a narcotic in a manner which deviates from accepted social and/or medical practices. However, Kanner and Foley feel that *addiction* is now preferably termed *psychological dependence,* which is a behavior pattern of compulsive drug use and preoccupation with securing its supply.

Kanner and Foley studied 86 cancer patients with carcinoma of the breast (34%), carcinoma of the lung (20%), tumors of the genitourinary system (14%), and various other malignancies. They felt that 62% of these patients had pain directly associated with tumor infiltration, 28% had pain from cancer therapy (radiation adhesions, etc), and 10% had pain unrelated to cancer. Kanner and Foley also studied 17 pain patients without cancer. Of the 103 patients studied, 65 were taking narcotics, 22 were not taking any analgesic, and five were taking aspirin or other non-narcotic analgesia. Eleven were taking other medications designed to help their pain (anticonvulsant, psychotropic, etc). Patients with tumor pain were found to take significantly higher doses of narcotics, and three patterns of drug use were noted.

The first group (14 patients) had doubled their narcotic use in a three-month follow-up period. Thirteen of the 14 had a malignant origin to their pain, and 12 of these 13 were dead at the six-month follow-up, due to their malignancy. Escalation of drug use was associated with rapidly progressing disease. A second group of 17 patients had no change in narcotic use and was found to have nonprogressive cancer, or a non-malignant pain syndrome. The third group of 14 patients either reduced (11/14) or stopped (3/14) narcotics. The reduction or cessation of narcotic use was related to concurrent anticancer therapy. Kanner and Foley concluded that increased narcotic use was associated with a worsening of cancer, while decreased use was associated with symptom improvement. They feel narcotics can be appropriately used in medically ill patients without a great risk of iatrogenic addictions.

Intellectual impairment as a side effect of narcotic administration had been advanced as a reason to eliminate narcotic use. However, in a study from Johns Hopkins Hospital by Hendler and his co-workers,[17] it was found that 35% of patients taking just narcotics have intellectual impairment, compared to 70% of the patients taking benzodiazepines (Librium, Valium, Dalmane, Tranxene, Ativan, Serax, etc). Rounsaville and his co-workers[18] at Yale evaluated 72 opiate addicts and compared them to 60 epilepsy patients, using finger tapping, pegboard, Trials A and B, visual search, color naming, H words, digit-symbol substitution, similarities, block design, and picture arrangement. These researchers found no difference between opiate addicts and epileptics when using these tests. Therefore, it seems that the degree of intellectual impairment due to narcotics is less than one may expect due to benzodiazepines, and may even be negligible.

With time contingency use of long-acting analgesic medications, it is possible to achieve a balance between the steady or continuous component of nociceptive input and blood level of analgesia with almost negligible side effects due to cerebral cortical intoxication. With prn or even regular use of short-acting agents, lasting usually two to three hours but given on a q4h basis, larger doses are necessary to achieve reasonable duration of action, and intervals of administration are kept longer than the duration of the desired analgesic effect in order to avoid respiratory depression.

REFERENCES

1. Black RG: The chronic pain syndrome. *Surg Clin North Am* 1975; 55:(4)999–1011.
2. Swerdlow M: The pain clinic. *Br J Clin Pract* 1972;26:403.
3. Ready LB, Black RG: Treatment of chronic pain with medications. (in press).
4. Sternbach RA: *Pain Patients, Traits and Treatment.* Academic Press, New York, 1974.
5. Hendler NH: The psychopharmacology of chronic pain, in *Diagnosis and Nonsurgical Management of Chronic Pain.* New York, Raven Press, 1981.
6. Fordyce WE: The office management of chronic pain. *Minn Med* 1974; 57:185–188.
7. Fordyce WE: Treating chronic pain by contingency management. *Adv Neurol* 1974;4:583–589.
8. Fordyce WE: *Behavioral Methods for Chronic Pain and Illness.* St Louis, CV Mosby Co, 1976.
9. Bonica JJ: *The Management of Pain.* Philadelphia, Lea & Febiger, 1953.
10. Foley KM: Pain syndromes in patients with cancer, in *Advances in Pain Research and Therapy.* New York, Raven Press, vol 2, 1979.
11. Loeser JD, Black RG: A taxonomy of pain. *Pain* 1975;1:81–84.
12. Lewis CS: *The Problem of Pain.* New York, Macmillan, 1973.
13. Sternbach RA: Strategies and tactics in the treatment of patients with pain, in *Pain and Suffering, Selected Aspects.* Springfield, Charles C Thomas, 1970, pp 176–185.
14. Merskey H: Psychological aspects of pain relief, in *Relief of Intractable Pain.* Amsterdam, Excerpta Medica, 1974, pp 90–115.
15. Melzack R, Torgerson WS: On the language of pain. *Anesthesiology* 1971;34:50–59.
16. Kanner RN, Foley KM: Patterns of narcotic drug use in a cancer pain clinic. Research developments in drug and alcohol use. *Ann NY Acad Sci* 1981;362:161–172.
17. Hendler N, Cimini C, Viernstein M, et al: A comparison of cognitive impairment due to narcotics and benzodiazepines. *Am J Psychiatry,* July 1980; 947–951.
18. Rounsaville B, Novelly R, Kleber H, et al: Neuropsychological impairment in opiate addicts: Risk factors. Research developments in drug and alcohol use. *Ann N Y Acad Sci* 1981;362:79–90.

20 Pastoral Care of the Chronic Pain Patient*

Chaplain, Major, Robert H. McPherson

The context of this presentation is a pain clinic or health care facility dedicated to holistic medicine where there is an open sharing of consult services. There is a trust in, knowledge of, and appreciation for the efforts other disciplines have in bringing relief to the suffering patient. In another setting, without this trust, some of the procedures set forth here may pose a threat to other health care professionals.

Pastoral care can be an integral part of interdisciplinary efforts to help the chronic pain patient. In an interdisciplinary approach to chronic pain, the boundaries between professional roles are fuzzy. Where do physical therapy, anesthesiology, orthopedics, neurosurgery, mental health, and neurology begin and leave off? Most of us know our own technical and ethical parameters and stay within them, but there is a merging of the circles of concern and practice when focused on the patient's needs.

The author does not write prescriptions, cut flesh, set bones, give shots, psychoanalyze, use hypnotherapy, or run electronic machinery used for diagnosis and treatment. Most health care professionals are not ordained by their religious body and do not serve communion, anoint the sick, hear confessions, pronounce absolution, or perform exorcisms on their patients. However, as a pastor, I often find myself using various techniques as a part of counseling which are also used by other disciplines: relaxation and breathing exercises in religious meditation, and the Gestalt method in counseling (particularly in working with grief).

I am overjoyed when other members of the health care team pray with their patients, refer to Scripture, and share their own therapeutic religious beliefs and convictions as they minister to the body and mind of their patients. This fulfills the Christian tradition of the priesthood of all believers. As a physician friend once said to me, "If you don't mind that I practice some good religion without ordination, I won't object if you practice some good medicine without licensure."

Religion and medicine have been linked together for thousands of years. In early civilizations, a shaman (a priest who cures the sick) was the only health care member of the tribe. Health and holiness were more than just semantically related. This was particularly true in the area of pain and suffering. It has only been within the last 200 years or so that pain was linked to any sensory perception.

Eastern religions view pain as ignorance; all passions are born of ignorance; the destruction of passions liberates one from suffering; liberation comes from ceasing to desire. Suffering results from wrong thinking and bad habits—not sin—just ignorance of the art of living.

The Old Testament is full of interpretations of pain and suffering. There seems to be a higher view of pain reflected as Jewish history and literature unfold. Even the casual reader of the Bible is aware of the several interpretations of personal pain:

- as a punishment for sin (Gen. 3, Job 4:8)
- as a chastening or disciplinary event (Prov. 3:11)
- as a testing by God (Prov. 3:11, Job 1:6–12)
- as a vicarious action on behalf of another (Isa. 53)
- as an event where God is a companion in suffering and ultimately the Savior (Mic. 4:10)

New Testament theology includes most of the interpretations given above, plus much more. Pain, in the Gospels and Epistles, is looked upon as a transforming event in the life of the person experiencing it, if this pain is offered to God or suffered on God's behalf. Because of pain, not in spite of it, a "gift" is received that otherwise may not have come.

Not that God sends the pain in order to make the gift possible, but God's omnipotence is shown as he uses pain and suffering and transforms it into an eternal gift. The crucifixion of Jesus is a case in point. Chronic pain can be approached on the same basis. Out of pain can emerge a saving grace.

Regardless of a patient's religious position, almost every person experiencing chronic pain becomes a philosopher or, more specifically, a theologian of sorts, seeking an ultimate explanation of suffering which will provide spiritual bracing for each new onslaught. Inner strength comes when one finds an adequate understanding of his suffering: when he knows from whence the pain comes and where he is going with it. If this internal strengthening is missing, the patient pulls down the flag of spiritual understanding, abandons the wheel of his ship of life and faith, and goes below, resigning the whole of life's enterprise to the storm.

The patient's theology becomes a life position which leads to growing health and wholeness or to continued illness and a worsening of "dis-ease." Theology determines to a large extent not only the nature but the duration of chronic pain. What the patient thinks about God probably affects how he interprets his pain and reacts to it and the means used to abate or remove it.

In order for a patient to make progress in dealing with chronic pain, he needs a relevant faith position in addition to an understanding of the physiological and psychological aspects of his illness and the therapeutic means used to aid in his recovery or management. The pastor's role in this regard is many faceted.

Pain may be abated or removed totally as spiritual therapies are introduced into the patient's life. I do not know why, but in some cases, through personal or intercessory prayer, laying on of hands, or anointing, pain is sometimes removed and even the biogenic cause taken away. This is always a possibility in these spiritual experiences. It has little to do with the religious background or even present state of the person's faith. God does not often act in this manner, but at times he does. I do not know why in many cases there is no removal or abatement, and in other cases there is relief. I only know that God remains the same and deals with us out of his pure love. As a pastor, I would want to lead my parishioner-patient toward this kind of spiritual understanding.

I also know that within the human body that God has created there are spiritual, chemical, and mental resources that can abate, remove, or help one to manage pain. We have much to learn here from the Eastern Christians. The fear or suspicion of Eastern religions, beliefs, and practices have caused many to purposely overlook or turn away from all the Eastern mind has to share. Westernized Christianity is long on outgoing pragmatism and short on getting in touch with the God within, long on product and short on process. We have concentrated too much on what we can get out of God and too little on getting to know God as he is and in listening to him. To do the latter takes discipline, effort, and training. It does not come overnight. It involves restructuring our cognitive and religious practices. Part of the work of a pastor working with chronic pain patients is educating the receptive patient in the art of prayer and meditation.

Often in the process of getting acquainted with the God within us, our pain response system is altered to the point that pain becomes manageable, but more importantly, the pain can be transformed and reveal a gift (deeper communion with life's source, greater compassion for man, new insight on life and death, revised plans, purposes, and priorities, new friendships, and new understandings and life styles for friends and loved ones).

As stated before, a patient who understands where his pain is coming from (etiology) and where he is creatively going with it (teleology) is in control of his life, even though the pain persists. My role as pastor is to be the living reminder of the faith by my presence, word, and deed.

Part of a patient's understanding is coming to terms with other factors present in his pain experience. Fear, anger, grief, and guilt are common casual or resultant elements in many chronic pain patients. Psychologists, psychiatrists, and other mental health professionals have made outstanding contributions in dealing with these "four horsemen" of chronic pain through individual and family counseling, hypnotherapy and psychoanalysis.

However, some patients are not interested in this approach and resent any inference, intended or not, by their physician that the "pain is in their head," they are manipulative, their marriage is in trouble, or they are seeking secondary gain. Any or all of these may be true. As a consequence, they may resist the valuable psychotherapeutic approach. Some of this antipathy to the psychological approach is reduced in an interdisciplinary setting since ideally all patients usually have thorough psychological testing, evaluation, and therapeutic recommendations or consultation as a part of their entrance to the program. Even then, some resistance may be encountered.

A trained clergyman, working in cooperation with the mental health department, can be of great assistance in removing some of the burden caused by anger, grief, guilt, and fear. Through Scripture, prayer, sacraments, rites, and personal counseling, fear can be replaced with trust in one's self, the health-care team, family, and God. Anger and guilt can be relieved through personal honesty, confession, and forgiveness. Grief can be assuaged through the facing of reality and encouragement to look toward the future with hope.

The pastoral counseling role is extremely valuable in helping the patient understand his illness, its affect on himself and others, and in reinforcing other behavioral science modes as part of a long-term rehabilitation program for chronic pain sufferers (biofeedback, contingency management, hypnotherapy, and analysis).

Another role of the pastor ministering to chronic pain patients is to direct them to the inner resources of their own faith. This can be done through various means, using some methods familiar to the patient, and introducing other forms that may be new.

If the patient has an active and wholesome life of prayer and biblical study, encouragement to continue in this manner is appropriate with perhaps little or no alteration in normal pattern and frequency. But many patients (perhaps even most) find prayer difficult and study out of the question.

> "I've prayed myself out. . . God doesn't seem to hear me. . . It's like I was talking to myself or to the walls. . . I'm not worthy. . . God must hate me for my sins. . . I hate God. . . Look what he has done to me. . . How much more does he expect me to take?. . . I feel embarrassed to call on God only when I need him. . . I haven't prayed before, except in Church and grace at meals. . . "

These are just a few of the many responses of pain patients which indicate that a patient has lost touch with his ability to communicate with God.

Even some who are praying regularly are in the very process of petition, focusing on their pain and furthering its continuance rather than receiving benefit. They have been praying their pain away for so long that prayer itself becomes a kind of reinforcer of their pain. Even the prayer, "God, help me to live with (cope with) this pain," becomes for some pain reinforcing, which sets a life-style centered on stoically dealing with pain, or pain becomes a way in which life or life with God is affirmed. Without pain there is death. Pain means life.

There are ways to break this cycle of nonproductive or counterproductive religious exercises and to introduce religious resources to the receptive patient.

If the patient has a church relationship where there are individuals or groups praying faithfully, I ask him to write or call that church and request that intercessory prayers be offered on his behalf. I also promise the patient that I, too, will pray for the relief of his pain, the wisdom to understand it, and the strength to work through it. I then ask the patient to stop praying for this matter of his personal pain (as much as humanly possible) for at least six weeks, trusting that others are praying for him and that God hears and answers their prayers.

I recommend that they adopt one or more of the following spiritual exercises which combine relaxation, breathing exercises, spiritual affirmations, assurances, teaching, and commitment. The goal of spiritual therapy is not to get immediate relief from the pain. In fact, there is no specific goal at all other than communion with God, no expectation, no manipulation of God or man through prayer. Simply stated, its only purpose is to center on God—his provision for every person's need, his grace, love, power, and hope—and let the other concerns of life be set aside during these moments.

Dr. Steven Brena, anesthesiologist and pain center director, in his book, *Pain and Religion*, sums up the thoughts of several mystics in these words:

> True prayer is not an action, but rather a listening in silence. It is not a message to be broadcast, but the joyous expectation of a divine Word to be revealed. It is not a list of needs and wants to be presented to God by beggars, but an act of knowledge and faith; the knowledge of our true identity and the faith that this knowledge will one day be transfigured into pure light, joy and bliss, the "Kingdom of God" in our hearts.

One of the easiest methods for Christian meditation is for the receptive patient to select a favorite Scripture passage or piece of liturgy (Lord's Prayer, Psalm 23, Apostles' Creed, or Rosary) which has been committed to memory or will be. Then set aside at least two 15 -minute periods for meditation during the day (the first thing in the morning and just before retiring). More time can be added as skill and comfortability increase. The novice may be able to do only five minutes or so at first, but later will increase the time to 15 or 20 minutes over a six-week period.

Once the passage is selected, the patient is asked to sit or be in as relaxed a position as possible. Most chronic pain patients have at least one pain free position. Then the patient is instructed to begin deep breathing and relaxation exercises until he feels as relaxed as possible. Continuing in this relaxed state, the person is asked to take the passage, one word or phrase at a time, and thoroughly ruminate that word or phrase in the mind and heart until all the meaning is drawn out. Then move on to the next word or phrase, continuing with the breathing exercises throughout the meditation, taking at least a deep breath and exhaling between each section. At the end of the passage, take two or three minutes of breathing exercise and then become alert and refreshed. This is not a novel procedure, but is similar to one encouraged by St. Theresa of Avila years ago and is described in her works, *The Way of Perfection and Internal Castles.*

The second method is to use prepared relaxation and meditative messages which are carefully read by a friend or relative, or using a cassette tape furnished by the pastor. The reading or recording is used two or three times during the day as a means of devotion which probably will be replaced in time by one's own memory or creative imagination.

The third method is to use an adaptation of the Eastern meditative Yoga technique. The patient selects a faith word or phrase (Jesus, Lord, *Maranantha, kurios,*) which has particular meaning or importance for him and on which he centers for 10 to 20 minutes. Again, as with the other two methods, there is no thought of this being used as a pain release mechanism—just clear communion with the inner reality of God. This is also combined with the disciplined breathing and relaxation techniques mentioned earlier. It differs from traditional transcendental meditation (TM), in that there is meaning in the word (or mantra); it has an origin in faith. Bodily posture is not rigidly defined, which would be difficult for most chronic pain patients at the beginning of their spiritual therapy. This is not to downgrade TM for there have been too many persons who have benefited from it to do that, but it is a less rigid procedure, is initiated personally, and has intentionality. That is, "centering prayer" has a goal, union and communion with God.

These are not new devices of Christian practice. They come down from the Eastern Christian tradition, from the fourth century monks of Egypt through St. Gregory of Sinai in the fourteenth century, and through one of the greatest spiritual fathers of the West, the twentieth-century Cistercian monk, Father Louis (Thomas) Merton. It is currently being used in many Christian communities throughout the world as a means to deepen spiritual life.

There is no gain or glory in pain itself; it contorts the face and isolates, vivid evidence that pain in itself is slow death. But the grace of Christ under the daily and mysterious overruling of God's providence can so change the spirit of the sufferer and so govern events that pain itself can become an open door to new life.

Suffering can be creative, depending on how we meet it and what we do with it. The Stoic accepts it with grim resolution and absorbs it. The Mohammedan says, "Kismet"—everything is the will of Allah and submits to it. The Buddhist turns the thought of it over in his mind and decides to evade it by escape to Nirvana. The Hindu traces it back to previous incarnations and sees it pursuing him in this and subsequent life and so feels the futility of submission, combat, or flight. The Old Testament righteous Jew considered that as long as he remained righteous, he was excused from it. But the Christian believes that pain can be used. He is not exempt from it, but when it comes he can use it to fertilize his character and to bring creative change and gifts into his life that otherwise would not have been present.

Great men and women, through pain, loneliness, and suffering throughout the ages, have brought forth some of the greatest literary, musical, and artistic works the world has seen or heard. The "average" man and woman, obscure and limited in experience and training, can also find that in their pain and suffering they can pipe their own personal songs, write their own intimate poetry, and paint their own masterpieces on the canvas of their lives.

Although this chapter is presented from the viewpoint of a Protestant pastor, the ideas and principles set forth are applicable, with some adaptation, to other faith groups.

BIBLIOGRAPHY

Bonica JJ: *The Management of Pain.* Philadelphia, Lea and Febiger, 1953.

Brena, S: *Pain and Religion. A Psychophysiological Study.* Springfield, IL, Charles C Thomas, 1972.

Crue BJ (ed): *Pain and Suffering. Selected Aspects.* Springfield, IL, Charles C. Thomas, 1970.

Diekman AJ: Implications of experimentally induced contemplative meditation. *J Nerv Ment Dis* 1966;142:101–116.

Fordyce WE: *Behavioral Methods for Chronic Pain and Illness.* St. Louis, Mosby, 1976.

Leroy PL (ed): *Current Concepts in the Management of Chronic Pain.* New York, Stratton Intercontinental Medical Book Corp, 1977.

Lewis CS: *The Problem of Pain.* London, Collins Press, 1961.

Meserve HD: Meditation and health. *J Rel Health* Spring 1980;19:No 1.

Pattison EM, Lapins NA, Doerr HA: Faith healing: A study of personality and function. *J Nerv Ment Dis* 1973;157:397–409.

Pennington MB: *Daily We Touch Him. Practical Religious Experience.* Garden City, NY, Doubleday and Co, Inc, 1977.

Weatherhead LP: *The Will of God.* Nashville, Abingdon Press, 1977.

APPENDIX

Possibilities for Pastoral Care Involvement In Pain Center/Clinic

As allowed by the patient, be a friend and pastor:

- another caring person (patient advocate role, as well)
- one whose role is familiar to patient

Counsel with patients during course of treatment regarding religious, spiritual, personal, or family concerns, carefully treating matters of pastoral privilege.

Develop and arrange for incoming interviews with pain patients based on the faith preference of the patient, obtaining, as appropriate, data related to the spiritual aspects (*pneumagenesis*) of the illness, i.e.:

- grief, loss, guilt, anxiety (religious, personal, family)
- "dis-ease" factors in illness, "anniversary reactions" to spirit affecting events

Direct patient to spiritual and faith resources for management of pain:

- deep spiritual meditation
- private devotional life
- pastoral counseling
- corporate worship, including sacramental resources (Holy Communion, anointing of the sick, healing services)
- church community resources

Be alert to patients on hospital wards and outpatients who may be in need of clinic/center services. (Be a public relations person for the center by interpreting program for patients.)

Informally obtain patients' reaction to their treatment, counsel in cases involving patient/staff relationships, and carry out follow-up visits.

Ministry to staff in pain center.

Occasional didactic presentation on relationship of stress to pain, attitudes, and religious resources.

Serve as a member of pain support group for inpatients and outpatients.

21 The Use of Physical Medicine and Rehabilitation in the Management of Pain

Marcel A. Reischer
Henry A. Spindler

The treatment modalities of physical medicine and rehabilitation are often useful in the management of both acute and chronic pain. These include various forms of rest, heat, cold, exercise, massage, traction, bracing, and electrical stimulation, as well as behavioral methods such as biofeedback, joint protection, and energy conservation for performing vocational and self-care activities. However, as with all other branches of medicine, consistently successful results with physical medicine require appropriate knowledge of the treatment modality used. These modalities have specific effects and side effects, indications, and contraindications. Heat may be useful in decreasing joint pain and stiffness in the arthritic, but may also increase joint swelling and enzymatic joint destruction. Cold may be used to decrease muscle spasm and pain, but may increase joint stiffness. Exercise may help strengthen or stretch weak, mechanically disadvantaged muscles but may irritate or excite trigger points and exacerbate joint pain. Rest may be useful in combating fatigue and joint pain but may lead to contractures, atrophy, and cardiovascular deconditioning.

Again, as with all other branches of medicine, accurate diagnosis is essential, both in terms of disease entity and structure involved as well as precipitating and aggravating factors. The physician must understand the disordered kinesiology and pathomechanics of the condition he is managing. Treatment of the painful low back without evaluation and treatment of predisposing causes of pelvic tilt (such as hamstring tightness and weak abdominal muscles) is often doomed to failure. Injecting an epicondylitis without subsequently stretching and strengthening the involved muscles is often inadequate. Managing a cervical radiculitis with the most sophisticated techniques available will be unsuccessful if one does not delve into the patient's work and personal history and investigate the causes and sources of chronic neck hyperextension. Individualization of the patient's program is critical. The treatment of a disorder in its chronic form is often quite different from treating the same disorder when seen acutely.

Treatment with physical medicine is generally by a team of professionals including physicians, physical therapists, occupational therapists, psychologists, social workers, and vocational counselors, as indicated. The physician must know what to expect of each of these professionals and what particular skill each has to offer to the patient. The role of physical therapy is familiar to most practitioners. They administer most of the previously mentioned modalities, as well as various exercises, and train the patient in ambulation and mobility. The role of the occupational therapist (OT) is often less well understood. The OT can also administer various forms of exercise but generally does this as part of a functional activity. This is often useful in patients who are resistant to participating in standard physical therapy programs. In addition, the OT is indispensable in helping the patient learn pain-saving and energy-saving techniques for self-care. Psychology is involved in counseling as well as the administration of biofeedback. Social service evaluation of the dynamics of the patient's home situation and vocational counseling are equally important in appropriate patients.

When prescribing a rehabilitation program, it is important to have specific goals and end points in mind. These end points should be realistic. It is often not appropriate to prescribe physical therapy for a patient who has chronic pain and not schedule a reevaluation until that patient has become totally asymptomatic. It is more appropriate to set realistic short-term goals in the hope of ultimately achieving the desired long-term goal, revising the program as the patient progresses. This approach allows the patient and the treating staff the possibility of positive reinforcement, and often helps break a vicious circle of pessimism that can be quite damaging to the patient and professional staff.

What follows is a brief description of some of the treatment modalities of physical medicine and rehabilitation. They can and should be used in various combinations, depending on the patient and problem. Again, the program should be individually tailored; routine prescriptions or protocols for pain patients are discouraged.

Rest

One of the most primitive, yet effective, modalities for pain relief is rest. Indeed, teleologically, one can conceive of protective muscle spasm as a splint to rest an affected part. It is the cornerstone of treatment of almost all acute musculoskeletal disorders, from fractures to muscle strains—literally from head to toe. Unfortunately, it is not without its complications. Among the most pernicious of these are muscle atrophy and weakness (it takes only half as long to lose muscular strength as it does to develop it) and the development of muscle tightness with consequently altered body mechanics. In the extreme, contractures can develop, which in themselves are painful and predispose to further pain as well. Loss of cardiovascular conditioning is well-documented and often limits the patient's ability to subsequently participate in an active rehabilitation program. Some of these complications can and should be prevented by awareness of their potential, as well as appropriate active and passive exercises in bed.

Therapeutic Heat

The local application of heat has been used for the relief of pain since antiquity. Analgesia and sedation are well-known effects of heat and are probably the result of a change in threshold perception of the free nerve endings. Muscle spasm is decreased by direct effects on the muscle spindles and gamma system. Heat causes an increase in extensibility of collagen tissue. This makes it most useful when treating contractures and muscle tightness and is one of the reasons that joint stiffness may be decreased with the use of heat. Heat often causes an increase in local blood flow, which is useful in the resolution of chronic inflammatory processes.

Heat also has side effects and contraindications. Increasing temperature increases the activity of proteolytic enzymes in rheumatoid arthritis and may accelerate the destructive process in the joints despite symptomatic improvement. Heat increases capillary dilatation and local blood flow, which often result in exacerbation of an acute inflammatory response, as well as increasing edema after acute injury. When extensive areas of the body are warmed, a generalized increase in cardiac output occurs. This can be dangerous in the patient with limited cardiovascular reserve. Local heat increases the metabolic demand of the tissue that it affects and, if there is inadequate circulation to that area due to vascular obstruction, may precipitate gangrene. Extreme care should be taken when treating patients with bleeding disorders or those who are anticoagulated, as the increased blood flow may lead to complications. Certainly heat is contraindicated in an area underlying suspected hemorrhage. Most heating modalities do not deliver precise amounts of heat, and generally require the patient's perception of warmth to prevent burns. Accordingly, heat is contraindicated in areas of decreased pain perception such as the extremities of individuals with peripheral neuropathies or following strokes with sensory impairment. Also, increasing body temperature such as after a whirlpool bath has been known to precipitate profound neurological deterioration in patients with multiple sclerosis.

Several forms of heat are available for treatment. Conductive heat transfer devices (electric heating pads, moist heat packs) and radiant heat (infrared lamp) are useful in providing heat to the skin and subcutaneous tissues. All have fundamentally the same effect, and the choice of modality often depends on patient and therapist preference. Patients often find it convenient to have their hands and wrists treated with paraffin which uniformly covers the part rather than with hot packs or radiant heat, which transfer their heat unevenly to such nonuniform surfaces. A whirlpool treatment is often very soothing, but the patient or therapist may not have the time for the preparation or cleanup that is necessary. Patients typically require 20 to 30 min of exposure to the superficial heating modality for good therapeutic effect to be noticed. It is very common in our experience for patients to be treated for inadequate periods of time, and this should be considered when patients have not done well with physical therapy.

Heat can also be delivered to tissues by conversion of electromagnetic energy through high-frequency electric currents (short-wave diathermy) or microwave radiation (microwave diathermy). High-frequency acoustical energy (ultrasound) can also be converted to heat. These techniques heat deeper structures than the conductive devices. Superficial muscle is best treated by short-wave diathermy and deeper muscles by microwave diathermy. Joint capsules and other deep structures, such as tendons, ligaments, and, occasionally, very deep muscles, are best treated by ultrasound. This group of modalities, in addition to the general complications of heat therapy, have their own set of unique problems. Short-wave diathermy, for example, cannot be used in the presence of metal implants or pacemakers, and microwave diathermy cannot be used near fluid-filled cavities (such as joint effusions) because of selective overheating of these structures.

Therapeutic Cold

The local application of cold has a number of beneficial therapeutic effects. Cold can produce pain relief by direct and indirect methods. Cold has effects similar to heat in blocking pain fiber transmission and altering pain threshold at free, nerve ending receptors. It is very effective in decreasing muscle spasm by altering spindle activity. Cold causes vasoconstriction which tends to limit an acute inflammatory response. On the other hand, cold reduces the distensibility of collagen which is probably, in part, responsible for the subjective complaints of increasing joint stiffness when arthritics are treated with cold. Contraindications to cold include cold hypersensitivity, Raynaud's phenomenon, cryoglobulinemia, and paroxysmal cold hemoglobinuria.

The techniques of cold application are not as sophisticated as those of therapeutic heat. Ice packs, cold wet packs, and various vapocoolant sprays (ethyl chloride, fluorimethane) are the methods generally used for administering cold. Skin, subcutaneous tissue, and superficial muscle can generally be affected by cold therapy. The extent and depth of cooling is dependent on the length of time the modality is in contact with the patient. Vapocoolant spray cooling is more dependent on the number of sweeps of spray over the treated area. Frostbite has rarely been reported when the patients have not been properly treated, so one should carefully observe the clinical response to cold. The initial skin analgesia may be useful, but the cooling of the underlying muscle may increase stiffness and be counterproductive. This is particularly important when treating myofascial syndromes with trigger points with the vapocoolant spray used as a means to ultimately increase tissue extensibility through allowing the patient to stretch them. If the vapocoolant spray is improperly administered, one may get a seemingly paradoxical effect.

Therapeutic Exercise

When prescribing exercise, the physician again must be certain what he is treating. There are various forms of exercise that are used in the treatment of pain. Patients who require primarily stretching exercises are often harmed by strengthening exercises. Patients who are treated with stretching exercises when their problems relate to decreased strength are often wasting their time. Again, careful assessment is critical prior to prescription.

Strengthening exercises can be isometric or isotonic. Both have been shown to effectively increase the strength of the exercised muscle group. Isometric exercises are useful in a patient with painful joints as they are performed without movement. They generally require less time to perform so that they can be more convenient for patients and therapists and also be useful for a patient as part of a home program. However, since most activities of daily living, including ambulation, require dynamic muscular activity, dynamic strengthening exercises should often be included in the program as well.

Strengthening exercises also have complications. Isometric exercise in particular should be used with caution in patients with cardiovascular disease and hypertension since it places an undue strain on the heart and circulation. Kinetic exercise performed too aggressively may exacerbate pain in a joint. "Overdoing it" may cause muscle pain and lead to further tightness of muscle and even to contractures.

For maximal effect the strengthening program should be carried out in a muscle of normal length. Unfortunately, many patients with acute pain and most with chronic pain have tightness of various muscle groups producing faulty biomechanics and predisposing to or indeed causing the patient's pain. One often cannot determine if the muscular weakness predisposed to the tightness or if the patient's faulty biomechanics caused the weakness. We tend, as a rule, to first treat the tightness and once improvement begins initiate appropriate strengthening exercises. Superficial heat or cold, and occasionally deep heat, are very useful prior to and during the stretching exercises as they decrease the patient's superficial pain; the deep heat increases the tissue extensibility. Other pain relieving techniques, such as transcutaneous electrical stimulation (TES), injections, or even pharmacological maneuvers, including oral and occasional parenteral analgesics and muscle relaxants, may be useful in enabling a patient to participate in an exercise program.

Massage

Massage is another well-known useful physical modality. Massage has a counterirritant effect which may help to alter the "reverberating circuit" of pain that often occurs. This may be its mode of action in relieving muscle spasm, something that it often does very effectively. Massage also stimulates the circulation locally, which may help "clean up" chronic inflammatory processes. It occasionally can be used to break adhesions between structures that cause pain and limit motion. It is often useful in relieving tension in the patient. It is not a substitute for exercise, although the relaxation and relief of spasm and pain one can achieve make it a useful adjunct to therapeutic exercise. There are some patients who simply cannot tolerate massage because of the tenderness of their muscles. The patients who have difficulty tolerating massage should be carefully examined for the presence of trigger points. Since massage may initiate pain in patients with trigger points, this modality is rarely useful for patients who harbor these.

Traction

Traction is one of the most overused, poorly prescribed physical medicine modalities. To have a distracting effect of the disc space and/or neural foramina, the force of traction must exceed the weight of the part being treated. In other words, to have a distracting effect cervical traction generally must be in the range of 25 pounds, and pelvic traction 80 to 100 pounds in the average patient. One must also remember that prior to distracting the intervertebral spaces the muscles, ligaments, fascia, joint capsules, and other soft tissues are usually stretched. This can also be done with less weight than is necessary to distract the spine. Stretching the soft tissues may be the mechanism by which traction helps some patients, particularly when inadequate forces for spinal distraction are applied. Soft tissue stretch, however, may also exacerbate the patient's pain, particularly if trigger points are present. Treatment of the patient's soft tissue disorder via trigger point injection, vapocoolant spray, stretch techniques, or other methods may be necessary prior to initiating cervical traction and relieving nerve root compression.

In addition to inadequate force, another common pitfall in administering traction is an improper angle of pull. Cervical spondylosis with radiculopathy is typically exacerbated by neck extension. Lumbosacral radiculopathies are also often exacerbated by extension of the back. One must be careful to inquire as to the angle of traction that was administered to a patient who experiences worsening of symptoms during the treatment. Pulling the neck or back into extension is, unfortunately, easy to do and commonly done. This is a particular problem with self-administered cervical traction that can be obtained through most surgical supply houses and many drugstores. Indeed, we see a number of patients whose symptoms have been primarily those of soft tissue restriction who were treated with home cervical traction, used the apparatus to promote neck extension, and consequently developed a cervical radiculopathy.

Electrotherapy

The pain-killing properties of electricity have been known since the days of the Romans, who used the electric eel for the treatment of headaches and gout. Electrical devices were used in quantity for numerous ailments at the turn of the century, but they fell into disrepute and were often considered quackery. In fact, however, therapeutic electricity has continued to be used for its effects of stimulating both innervated and denervated muscle. Widespread use of TENS (discussed elsewhere in this book) has spurred a resurgence of interest in electrotherapy. The TENS device is a relatively low voltage stimulator with a primary effect of blocking pain transmission. TENS does nothing about the cause of pain. Electrical stimulation of muscle does have a very definite effect on the muscle and is used for these effects rather than for analgesia. Over the past few years, a number of manufacturers have developed higher voltage galvanic and faradic stimulators with the capability of stimulating the neuromuscular apparatus. These are often useful in the treatment of acute muscle spasm where a tetanizing stimulation ultimately fatigues and relaxes the muscle, enabling the muscle to be stretched. This often results in marked pain relief in the acute stages of pain. Our results with chronic pain are less encouraging, perhaps because what is considered to be muscle spasm in chronic myofascial syndromes is often a chronically contracted muscle associated with edema and fibrosis. In the acute muscle spasm, increased muscular activity can be recorded by electromyographic techniques. In the patient with chronic pain, electrodiagnostic studies indicate a marked reduction in actual muscular activity despite a clinical "spasm" on inspection and palpation.

Braces

Braces can be used to stabilize, immobilize, or support painful structures. Progressive casting can correct a deformed and contracted joint. There are literally dozens of different neck and back braces available. In the patient without fractures, we find that a simple lumbosacral corset is as effective as any other brace for acute or chronic low back pain. It acts primarily by giving support to the abdominal muscles and to a lesser extent, reinforcing the lumbosacral spine extensors. It is easily cared for by the patient and is inconspicuously worn. It does not adequately immobilize the spine, and if this effect is specifically desired, the stronger but more cumbersome and more poorly tolerated braces should be tried. Braces tend to make the patient use his muscles less, thereby leading to weakening of those muscles. Strengthening exercises for the trunk muscles should always be considered in conjunction with bracing.

A properly fitted, soft cervical collar is generally all that is needed for patients with cervical spondylosis. This reminds the patient to voluntarily restrict his painful motion and, in most patients, it should fasten in the front to allow flexion but limit extension. When properly fitted, a soft cervical collar supports the head and allows the neck muscles to rest, which also contributes to pain relief. This type of collar is often worn by victims of motor vehicle accidents, and, indeed, patients often call these "whiplash collars." Unlike lumbosacral supports, which cannot be seen when worn, a cervical collar can. It may evoke sympathy from family and friends, thereby providing secondary gain for the patient. Conversely, cynicism may greet the patient with a collar, and the patient may have to resort to more extensive acting out to get appropriate attention.

For these reasons, as well as the development of muscle weakness and possibly decreased range of motion, we try to have our patients wear these devices for as short a time as possible.

Braces and splints are often useful in other conditions as well. Carpal tunnel syndrome can often be managed conservatively by using a wrist splint that prevents wrist flexion. Patients with chronic tennis elbow may find a splint that prevents active wrist extension useful. Splints are also available that limit the excursion of the muscles that are involved in this condition. Knee and ankle braces may provide added support in patients with disorders in this area. One should be wary, however, of the development of patellofemoral problems secondary to the compression of the brace.

Joint and Energy Conservation: Activities of Daily Living

This is one of the most important yet most overlooked functions of the rehabilitation team. Despite all of the modalities of treatment described in this book, many patients continue to have pain. Training in appropriate modifications of self-care techniques can often make a remarkable difference in the quality of the patient's life. Assistive devices such as elevated toilet seats and tub benches allow the patient to do activities that their stiff painful joints and weak extremities would not allow them to do previously. Reachers of various sorts allow the patient to dress the lower extremities where the back and lower extremity joints did not allow it previously. Appropriate modifications often can be made inexpensively to the kitchen and help the patient resume functioning in that setting. A wheeled cart for carrying heavy items is often very useful. Proper techniques for bending and lifting are critical for the patient with chronic pain to learn. Training in organizing one's day is very important for the patient with limited mobility and endurance. Evaluation of the patient's activities of daily living is generally best performed by an occupational therapist. A rehabilitation nurse and physical therapist may be helpful as well.

Conclusions

Those of us who frequently see patients who are referred for evaluation of chronic pain syndrome find that these patients have often already been through several long, painful, expensive, and ineffective physical therapy programs and are resistant to even attempting further treatment. It is important for all to realize that the patient's failure to respond to therapy may have been related to misdiagnosis, use of an incorrect heating modality with inappropriate depth of penetration or inadequate duration of exposure, use of the wrong exercise at the wrong time, or any other of the common pitfalls. Accurate diagnosis is essential, as is goal-oriented treatment. Effective physical treatment may require the adjunctive use of nonphysical measures such as injections or medicinal analgesics. Frequent evaluation is essential. Acute pain can often be transformed into chronic pain with all of its attendant implications during the course of physical treatment. Reevaluations are essential to determine the patient's response to the treatment and the reasons for lack of response. It has been said, "If acute pain were approached more astutely, there would be less chronic pain." To be sure, this applies as much to the use of physical medicine and rehabilitation methods as it does to any other medical and allied health professional intervention.

BIBLIOGRAPHY

Basmajian JV: *Therapeutic Exercise,* ed 3. Baltimore, Williams and Wilkins 1978.

Cailliet R: *Soft Tissue Pain and Disability.* Philadelphia, FA Davis, 1977.

Krusen FH, Kottke FJ, Ellwood PM: *Handbook of Physical Medicine and Rehabilitation,* ed 2. Philadelphia, WB Saunders, 1971.

Physiatric Therapeutics, MKSAP in Physical Medicine and Rehabilitation Syllabus. Chicago, American Academy of Physical Medicine and Rehabilitation, 1977.

INDEX